"Rienecke and Le Grange present a scholarly synthesis of research on expressed emotion in families – a critical factor in many forms of psychopathology including eating disorders. Expressed emotion is a demonstrated moderator of treatment outcomes as well as a variable worthy of intervention efforts in its own right. From the origins of the study of expressed emotion to recent, novel applications and emerging new findings, this book represents a definitive compilation on the topic that is essential for the libraries of clinicians and researchers alike."

Katharine L. Loeb, PhD, Professor of Psychology, PhD Program in Clinical Psychology, Fairleigh Dickinson University

"In this volume, Drs. Rienecke and Le Grange provide an essential examination of the concept of expressed emotion among individuals with eating disorders and their family members. Chapters authored by research and clinical experts systematically disentangle the complexity of expressed emotion through comprehensive literature reviews, rich case examples, and innovative theoretical conceptualizations. State-of-the-art information about cultural influences, measurement considerations, treatment approaches, and research priorities deepen the reader's understanding of these interactional patterns as well as the importance of contextual factors. An extremely valuable resource, this book provides a critical perspective to understanding relational aspects of eating disorders that can help guide us toward effective interventions for those suffering from eating disorders and their families."

Carol B. Peterson, PhD, Associate Professor of Psychiatry, University of Minnesota

"Despite recent advances in our knowledge and understanding of the role of Expressed Emotion (EE) in the field of eating disorders, gaps unfortunately remain. Like never before, this group of eminent scientists and clinicians have shared their collective knowledge and experience to produce a very valuable book. Where this book comes into its own, is its aim to further our understanding of EE from both a scholarly and clinical perspective. It is clearly and concisely written and is full of valuable clinical advice. This book is a must read for researchers and clinicians alike, and I have little doubt that it will stimulate much needed innovative research in this domain in the years to come."

Stephen W. Touyz, PhD, Professor Emeritus, School of Psychology and Inside Out Institute, University of Sydney

Eating Disorders and Expressed Emotion

The first to synthesize the exponentially growing research on expressed emotion (EE) and eating disorders and apply it to treatment, interventions, and other scenarios, this unique text provides unprecedented guidance to students, clinicians, and researchers in the field of eating disorders.

This book explores the components of relatives' attitudes and behaviors toward an ill family member and discusses a modifiable treatment target that could improve outcomes for patients through interventions, treatment plans, and future directions in research. Chapters bring together contributions from eminent scientists and clinicians in the fields of families, eating disorders, and treatment to contribute to the clinical and scholarly understanding of expressed emotion and eating disorders.

Mental health professionals studying and treating eating disorders will find this text to be a valuable reference guide and will be inspired to further explore this rich and promising area of study.

Renee D. Rienecke, PhD, FAED, is Director of Research for Eating Recovery Center/Insight Behavioral Health Centers and Associate Professor in the Department of Psychiatry and Behavioral Sciences at Northwestern University.

Daniel Le Grange, PhD, FAED, is a Benioff UCSF Professor of Children's Health and Director of the Eating Disorders Program in the Department of Psychiatry at the University of California, San Francisco. Dr. Le Grange is also Emeritus Professor of Psychiatry and Behavioral Neuroscience at the University of Chicago.

Eating Disorders and Expressed Emotion

Integrating Treatment, Intervention, and a Positive Family Environment

Edited by
Renee D. Rienecke and Daniel Le Grange

Routledge
Taylor & Francis Group
NEW YORK AND LONDON

First published 2021
by Routledge
52 Vanderbilt Avenue, New York, NY 10017

and by Routledge
2 Park Square, Milton Park, Abingdon, Oxon, OX14 4RN

Routledge is an imprint of the Taylor & Francis Group, an informa business

Library of Congress Cataloging-in-Publication Data
Names: Rienecke, Renee D. (Renee Dawn), editor. | Le Grange, Daniel, editor.
Title: Eating disorders and expressed emotion : integrating treatment, intervention, and a positive family environment / edited by Renee D. Rienecke, Daniel Le Grange.
Description: New York, NY : Routledge, 2020. | Includes bibliographical references and index.
Identifiers: LCCN 2020005282 (print) | LCCN 2020005283 (ebook) | ISBN 9781138367968 (hardback) | ISBN 9781138367982 (paperback) | ISBN 9780429429484 (ebook)
Subjects: MESH: Feeding and Eating Disorders—psychology | Expressed Emotion | Feeding and Eating Disorders—therapy | Family Relations—psychology | Psychosocial Support Systems
Classification: LCC RC552.E18 (print) | LCC RC552.E18 (ebook) | NLM WM 175 | DDC 616.85/26—dc23
LC record available at https://lccn.loc.gov/2020005282
LC ebook record available at https://lccn.loc.gov/2020005283

ISBN: 978-1-138-36796-8 (hbk)
ISBN: 978-1-138-36798-2 (pbk)
ISBN: 978-0-429-42948-4 (ebk)

Typeset in Adobe Caslon Pro
by Apex CoVantage, LLC

RDR: To my parents, Evon and Rick, and to Jan.

DLG: This book is for Zoë, her mother, late grandmother, and great grandmother.

Contents

List of Figures xi
List of Tables xii
List of Contributors xiii

1 Introduction to the Construct of Expressed Emotion 1
Renee D. Rienecke and Daniel Le Grange

2 Expressed Emotion and Psychosis 7
Juliana Onwumere and Elizabeth Kuipers

3 Beneath the Surface of Expressed Emotion (EE): The Clinical Relevance of Possible Mechanisms Underlying EE in Eating Disorders 33
Mima Simic, Tom Jewell, and Ivan Eisler

4 Assessment of Expressed Emotion 58
Erica Allan, Renee D. Rienecke, and Elizabeth K. Hughes

5 Expressed Emotion and Anorexia Nervosa 76
Sasha Gorrell and Daniel Le Grange

6 Expressed Emotion and Bulimia Nervosa 101
Renee D. Rienecke

7 Emotionally Driven Behaviors (Expressed Emotion, Accommodating, Enabling, and Splitting) and How to Manage Them in the Social Network of People With Eating Disorders 115
Janet Treasure, Dan Willmott, and Valentina Cardi

8 Cultural Differences in Expressed Emotion 129
Tecelli Domínguez-Martínez and Cristina Medina-Pradas

9 Factors Associated With High Expressed Emotion Versus Low Expressed Emotion 156
Kathryn M. Huryk and Eric F. van Furth

10 Future Directions in Expressed Emotion 176
Renee D. Rienecke and Gina Dimitropoulos

Index 187

Figures

3.1 Theoretical model for role of high expressed emotion in the eating disorder treatment process 44
7.1 The interpersonal element of the cognitive interpersonal model 117

TABLES

7.1 The reaction of close others to ED behaviors 117
7.2 Caregiving behaviors to be increased 123
7.3 Theories and strategies to moderate maladaptive interpersonal reactions 123
8.1 Descriptive data of patients, carers, and EE scores from the 18 studios selected by Anastasiadou et al. (2014), including new information of place of study and ethnic group of samples 142

CONTRIBUTORS

Erica Allan is a psychologist within the Eating Disorders Service at The Royal Children's Hospital, Australia. Her area of clinical interest and practice is focused on restrictive eating disorders. She has previously worked as a research assistant at the Royal Children's Hospital Eating Disorders Service before completing her clinical training.

Valentina Cardi, PhD is a clinical psychologist specialized in the assessment and treatment of individuals with eating disorders. She is currently a Lecturer at King's College London, and her research focuses on the development and evaluation of treatment enhancers to improve the outcomes of standard interventions for eating disorders. Dr. Cardi is particularly interested in the use of novel technologies to deliver psychological treatment.

Gina Dimitropoulos is Associate Professor in the Faculty of Social Work, University of Calgary. She has over 20 years of clinical experience in both tertiary care and community-based settings delivering family-based treatments, group therapy, and individual counseling for adolescents and adults with eating disorders. She is also the research lead for the Calgary Eating Disorder Program, where she is overseeing research in family-based treatment for adolescents and emerging adults with eating disorders.

Tecelli Domínguez-Martínez, PhD received her PhD in clinical and health psychology at the University Autonomous of Barcelona (Spain). Dr. Domínguez-Martínez is currently a medical science researcher at the Research Center on Global Mental Health, Direction of Epidemiology and Psychosocial Research, "Ramón de la Fuente Muñiz" National Institute of Psychiatry in Mexico City. Her research focuses on psychosocial risk factors, diagnosis, classification, early detection and intervention in severe mental disorders, family environment, and family factors in the development and course of mental disorders, including the study of expressed emotion in the early stages of psychosis. Furthermore, Dr. Domínguez-Martínez has worked on multiple field studies of the World Health Organization to validate the Mental and Behavioural Disorders chapter from the Eleventh Revision of the International Classification of Diseases and Related Health Problems (ICD-11).

Ivan Eisler, OBE, PhD, FAcSS, FAED, is joint head of the Maudsley Centre for Child and Adolescent Eating Disorders at the South London and Maudsley NHS Foundation Trust and Emeritus Professor at Kings College London. He is known as a leading developer and researcher of evidence-based psychotherapies for eating disorders, including single and multifamily therapy for eating disorders (aka "Maudsley Family Therapy") and has played a key role in the development of dedicated community-based eating disorders services for children and adolescents across England. He has also contributed to treatment research for other disorders such as adolescent self-harm, depression, substance misuse, and conduct disorder.

Sasha Gorrell, PhD is a NIMH-funded T32 postdoctoral research scholar in the Eating Disorders Program at the University of California, San Francisco, mentored by Daniel Le Grange, PhD. She earned her PhD in clinical psychology from the University at Albany in 2018, where her graduate research included a pilot intervention promoting healthy eating and exercise behavior among female professional ballet dancers. The overarching goal of her research is to better understand the use of adaptive and maladaptive strategies for the self-regulation of weight, including biobehavioral processes contributing to reward learning and engagement in unhealthy exercise behaviors.

Elizabeth K. Hughes, PhD is a research fellow at the University of Melbourne and Murdoch Children's Research Institute, Australia. She has led research and service evaluation at the Melbourne Royal Children's Hospital Eating Disorders Service for the past ten years with a focus on family-based treatment (FBT) for adolescents with anorexia nervosa and other restrictive eating disorders. Dr. Hughes has published widely on adaptations to FBT, treatment implementation and outcomes, and eating disorder symptoms in population-based cohorts. Her research interests also include psychiatric comorbidity in eating disorders, body image, emotion regulation, and family systems.

Kathryn M. Huryk, MA, is a predoctoral clinical psychology fellow in the Eating Disorders Program at University of California, San Francisco, and a doctoral candidate at Fairleigh Dickinson University. She graduated from Barnard College with a BA in psychology and English. Kathryn has received extensive clinical training in evidence-based assessment and intervention across a wide range of settings, including the Eating Disorders Center at New York–Presbyterian Hospital and the Anxiety and Mood Program at Montefiore Medical Center. Her research focuses on the prevention and treatment of eating disorders in children and adolescents.

Tom Jewell, MSc, BSc, RMN, is a family therapist and mental health nurse, currently completing a NIHR Clinical Doctoral Fellowship at King's College London. He works clinically at the Maudsley Centre for Child and Adolescent Eating Disorders. His PhD is investigating attachment and mentalization as predictors of outcome in family therapy for adolescent anorexia nervosa.

Elizabeth Kuipers, OBE, is Professor Emerita of Clinical Psychology at the Institute of Psychiatry, Psychology and Neuroscience (IoPPN), King's College London. Professor Kuipers has authored and co-authored more than 400 articles, book chapters, and books and has more than 15,000 citations for her work. She was the chair of the National Institute of Health and Clinical Excellence (NICE) Psychosis and Schizophrenia updated treatment Guideline for England and Wales in 2014 and

2009. She is a fellow of the British Psychological Society and recipient of two Lifetime Achievement Awards. In 2018, as part of the New Year Honours List, Elizabeth was awarded an OBE for services to psychosis research, treatment, and care.

Daniel Le Grange, PhD, FAED, is a Benioff UCSF Professor of Children's Health and director of the Eating Disorders Program in the Department of Psychiatry at the University of California, San Francisco. Dr. Le Grange is also Emeritus Professor of Psychiatry and Behavioral Neuroscience at the University of Chicago.

Cristina Medina-Pradas, PhD, is Associate Professor in the Department of Psychology at International University of La Rioja and researcher within the Mental Problems and Social Dysfunctions Team of the Department of Personality, Assessment, and Psychological Treatments at University of Seville (Spain). Dr. Medina-Pradas also serves as a coordinator of a regional psychotherapeutic program aimed toward children and mothers who have suffered gender violence at the perinatal stage and who attend her clinical consultation in Seville. Dr. Medina-Pradas has done extensive research on interviewing and assessment techniques for working with families of psychosis, eating disorders, and other psychiatric patients and has been actively involved in research on the influence of family expressed emotion on psychiatric illness for more than 15 years. Her work has focused on psychopathology, psychotic continuum, at-risk mental states, prevention, psychosocial factors, emotions, family and stress, and perinatal psychology.

Juliana Onwumere, PhD is Senior Lecturer in the Department of Psychology at the Institute of Psychiatry, Psychology and Neuroscience, King's College London. She is a consultant clinical psychologist with the National Psychosis Unit and the Psychological Interventions Clinic for Outpatients with Psychosis at the South London and Maudsley NHS Foundation Trust in London. Her research and clinical interests are focused on family issues in psychosis, particularly improving the development, training, and wider provision of cognitive behavioral therapy for psychosis, and family interventions. She developed the first international massive open online course on caring for people with psychosis and schizophrenia. Dr. Onwumere has authored several academic papers and book chapters on family-related issues in psychosis.

Renee D. Rienecke, PhD, FAED, is Director of Research for Eating Recovery Center/Insight Behavioral Health Centers and Associate Professor in the Department of Psychiatry and Behavioral Sciences at Northwestern University. She has over 20 years of experience in the treatment of eating disorders, particularly in family-based treatment, and has built and developed two eating disorder programs at the University of Michigan and at the Medical University of South Carolina. Her research interests include the role of expressed emotion in treatment outcome for adolescent anorexia nervosa and bulimia nervosa.

Mima Simic, MD, MSc, MRCPsych, is joint head of the Maudsley Centre for Child and Adolescent Eating Disorders and a consultant child and adolescent psychiatrist at the South London and Maudsley NHS Foundation. She led the development of intensive treatment programs for eating disorders that offer an integrative approach combining family therapy, multi-family therapy, dialectical behavior therapy, and radical openness for adolescent therapy interventions. Dr. Simic has also contributed to research studies ranging from neuroimaging studies of adolescent depression and anorexia nervosa to testing manualized treatments in eating disorders and self-harm.

Janet Treasure, MD, PhD completed her medical degree and a PhD in physiology at St. Thomas' Medical School. She then did her clinical training as a physician and a psychiatrist. For much of her career, Dr. Treasure has specialized in the treatment of eating disorders at the Maudsley Hospital and in King's College London. She has carried out extensive research – often collaboratively with patients and carers – that has led to greater understanding of and better treatments for eating disorders. Dr. Treasure has trained over 40 PhD students, who have implemented various aspects of translational psychiatry as part of their research training. Many of them have progressed to hold important academic and clinical positions in eating disorders. She has worked collaboratively with other international centers. In total, she has authored more than 600 scientific articles. As well as writing professional texts, Dr. Treasure has co-produced self-care interventions (in books and e-health formats) for people affected by eating disorders and their carers. She has received many awards for her research. In 2012, she was awarded an OBE for her work with people with eating disorders.

Eric F. van Furth, PhD, FAED, is the director at GGZ Rivierduinen Eating Disorders Ursula, an eating disorder center of excellence in Leiden, the Netherlands. He is Professor of Eating Disorders in the Department of Psychiatry, Leiden University Medical Center. Dr. van Furth is a clinical psychologist and family therapist. After receiving his PhD in psychology from Utrecht University, van Furth went on to pen more than 90 publications, primarily journal articles, chapters, educational videos, and conference papers, on eating disorders. He has also published three books on the subject and is a member of the editorial advisory boards of the *International Journal of Eating Disorders*, *European Eating Disorders Review*, and *Eating Behaviors*. He has been working clinically with patients with eating disorders for more than 35 years. He is currently the president of the Dutch Academy for Eating Disorders. Last, Dr. van Furth is a fellow and past president of the Academy for Eating Disorders.

Dan Willmott completed his undergraduate psychology BSc and cognitive neuroscience MSc at the University of Sussex, where he worked within the Sackler Centre for Consciousness Science researching the interactions between the heart and the brain, specifically, how interoceptive processes influence fear learning. Dan then completed further clinical training at King's College London and worked within a child and adolescent counseling service as a Wellbeing Practitioner. Dan has extensive interest in eating disorders, having provided support to people with eating disorders within his personal life. Dan is currently managing a large clinical trial testing how the provision of online support to patients with anorexia nervosa and their carers can improve outcomes in those with a severe and enduring form of the illness.

1

Introduction to the Construct of Expressed Emotion

Renee D. Rienecke and Daniel Le Grange

Introduction

Expressed emotion (EE) was first conceptualized in the 1950s by George Brown, a British sociologist, and his colleagues while studying patients with schizophrenia. They observed that patients who were discharged from an inpatient unit to live with their parents or spouses relapsed at significantly higher rates in the first year after discharge than did patients who lived with siblings or in lodgings away from their families (Brown, Carstairs, & Topping, 1958). This led to an exploration of different aspects of family life that could account for this finding. A study of 128 men with a diagnosis of schizophrenia found that 76% of patients returning to "high emotional involvement" homes (defined then as homes with relatives showing "strongly expressed emotion", hostility, or dominating behavior) deteriorated in the first year after discharge from the hospital compared with 28% who returned to "low emotional involvement" homes (Brown, Monck, Carstairs, & Wing, 1962). These findings remained even when symptom severity at time of discharge was accounted for. Results were replicated in a later study, and the term "expressed emotion" was introduced (Brown, Birley, & Wing, 1972).

EE was originally measured with an interview that could take four or five hours to administer (Brown & Rutter, 1966; Rutter & Brown, 1966). To counter this time-consuming process, Christine Vaughn and Julian

Leff were instrumental in developing the Camberwell Family Interview (CFI). Contrary to its name, this interview of a caregiver about their unwell relative was shorter and more manageable to administer and score, further facilitating the study of EE (Vaughn & Leff, 1976a). As a result, EE is now known to play an important role in the outcome of a range of disorders, including depression (Uehara, Yokoyama, Goto, & Ihda, 1996; Vaughn & Leff, 1976b), anxiety (Chambless & Steketee, 1999; Garcia-Lopez, Muela, Espinosa-Fernandez, & Diaz-Castela, 2009), eating disorders (Duclos, Vibert, Mattar, & Godart, 2012; Rienecke, 2018), diabetes (Liakopoulou et al., 2001), and epilepsy (Bressi et al., 2007).

Briefly returning to EE's founding father, Brown et al. (1972) established that the number of Critical Comments made by the ill relative's caregiver was the single most important factor contributing to the overall level of EE. This, along with a relative lack of research on warmth and positive remarks has led to EE taking on a largely negative connotation over the years. However, Brown's intention was not to uncover pathological family functioning but to identify attitudes and behaviors found in "ordinary families" (Leff & Vaughn, 1985) and to avoid blaming families for any worsening of symptoms seen in their ill relatives. Even in the 1950s, when the concept of a "schizophrenogenic mother" was popular, Brown cautioned against blaming parents:

> Even if differences exist between the mothers of schizophrenics and other mothers, this need not be of aetiological importance. The possibility must first be excluded that behavior such as "overprotectiveness" may be the result of the patient's unusual behavior influencing the parents.
>
> (Brown et al., 1962, p. 55)

Thus, it is important to emphasize that EE does not "blame" caregivers for causing psychiatric illnesses; instead, it focuses on factors influencing the course of illness (Brown et al., 1972). Brown's view is similar to that of Whitney and Eisler (2005), who suggested that when families are faced with the stresses of a member with a potentially life-threatening illness, such as an eating disorder, their internal resources and strengths can be negatively impacted. This, in turn, can lead to family interactions that maintain, rather than challenge, the eating disorder. This is also in line with views about the direction of causality in EE, which has been a matter of some debate in the field (King, 2000; Leff, 1989). Does high EE, on the part of the parent, lead to poor outcome and relapse, or does problematic behavior on the part of the patient, such as poor response to treatment, lead to the development of high parental EE? It has been suggested that some degree of circular interaction is likely taking place (Hooley & Richters, 1995; Leff, 1989), with each influencing the other over time. Although caregivers may inadvertently behave in ways that can maintain symptoms over time, EE has been found to be a modifiable factor in the field of schizophrenia (Öksüz, Karaca, Özaltin, & Ateş, 2017). There also is limited evidence that some interventions to reduce EE have been successful in the field of eating disorders (Hibbs et al., 2015; Uehara, Kawashima, Goto, Tasaki, & Someya, 2001). Thus, the study of EE has provided us with a treatment target, one that can ultimately improve treatment outcome for patients.

Over the years, the assessment of EE has also provided us with a rich source of clinical information for our work with families and a growing body of research that has advanced our understanding of the role of EE in eating disorders. This book has brought together some of the premier researchers in the field of EE and eating disorders to synthesize this literature and identify areas for future research that can improve our understanding of this important construct. The book begins by placing EE in its historical context by reviewing its development in the field of psychosis, discussing EE in the caregiving relationship, and outlining ways in which high EE can be addressed in both individual and family work by presenting three case descriptions (Chapter 2; Onwumere & Kuipers). This chapter sets the stage for the examination of EE in the context of eating disorders, beginning with an explanation of why it is an important domain to study. This is followed by an overview of the literature on EE and eating disorders and the proposition of a neurobiologically informed theory that considers temperament, cognitive appraisal and emotion regulation – a theory that may serve to deepen our understanding of EE and guide future research efforts (Chapter 3; Simic, Jewell, & Eisler). Chapter 4 (Allan, Rienecke, & Hughes) reviews what is assessed when rating each subscale of EE and outlines the various ways in which EE can be measured. Since the development of what is often considered the "gold-standard" assessment interview, the CFI (Vaughn & Leff, 1976a), other, briefer measures have been developed that contributed to a more widespread study of EE, although at the same time perhaps sacrificing some of the rich clinical data provided by the CFI. This chapter is followed by comprehensive reviews of EE in anorexia nervosa (AN) and bulimia nervosa (BN) in Chapters 5 (Gorrell & Le Grange) and 6 (Rienecke) respectively, as these are the two eating disorders that have been studied most extensively in the context of EE. Managing a variety of emotionally driven behaviors, including EE, among caregivers of those with eating disorders is addressed in the context of the cognitive-interpersonal model of AN (Chapter 7; Treasure, Willmott, & Cardi) followed by an area of EE that is particularly under-researched, i.e., cultural differences in EE (Chapter 8; Domínguez-Martínez & Medina-Pradas). EE is a highly cultural construct, and it is useful to have an understanding of a family's cultural and ethnic background before attempting to rate the family's level of EE. Family and patient factors associated with high versus low EE are reviewed by Huryk and van Furth (Chapter 9). A number of factors have been shown to differentiate parents who are low or high on EE, including caregiver burden, psychological distress, carer coping, attributional style, and gender. This edited volume concludes with the identification and discussion of future areas for research in EE and eating disorders (Chapter 10; Rienecke & Dimitropoulos).

EE has been found to be a consistent prognostic indicator for a wide range of disorders and has remained an important and relevant construct for half a century. With this book, we and our colleagues hope to contribute to the clinical and scholarly understanding of EE and eating disorders and stimulate much needed work in this domain.

References

Bressi, C., Cornaggia, C. M., Beghi, M., Porcellana, M., Iandoli, I. I., & Invernizzi, G. (2007). Epilepsy and family expressed emotion: Results of a prospective study. *Seizure*, *16*, 417–423.

Brown, G. W., Birley, J. L. T., & Wing, J. K. (1972). Influence of family life on the course of schizophrenic disorders: A replication. *British Journal of Psychiatry*, *121*, 241–258.

Brown, G. W., Carstairs, G. M., & Topping, G. (1958). Post-hospital adjustment of chronic mental patients. *Lancet*, *272*, 685–689.

Brown, G. W., Monck, E. M., Carstairs, G. M., & Wing, J. K. (1962). Influence of family life on the course of schizophrenic illness. *British Journal of Preventive & Social Medicine, 16*, 55–68.

Brown, G. W., & Rutter, M. (1966). The measurement of family activities and relationships: A methodological study. *Human Relations, 19*, 241–263.

Butzlaff, R. L., & Hooley, J. M. (1998). Expressed emotion and psychiatric relapse: A meta-analysis. *Archives of General Psychiatry, 55*, 547–552.

Chambless, D. L., & Steketee, G. (1999). Expressed emotion and behavior therapy outcome: A prospective study with obsessive-compulsive and agoraphobic outpatients. *Journal of Consulting and Clinical Psychology, 67*, 658–665.

Duclos, J., Vibert, S., Mattar, L., & Godart, N. (2012). Expressed emotion in families of patients with eating disorders: A review of the literature. *Current Psychiatry Reviews, 8*, 183–202.

Garcia-Lopez, L. J., Muela, J. M., Espinosa-Fernandez, L., & Diaz-Castela, M. (2009). Exploring the relevance of expressed emotion to the treatment of social anxiety disorder in adolescence. *Journal of Adolescence, 32*, 1371–1376.

Hibbs, R., Magill, N., Goddard, E., Rhind, C., Raenker, S., Macdonald, P., . . . Treasure, J. (2015). Clinical effectiveness of a skills training intervention for caregivers in improving patient and caregiver health following in-patient treatment for severe anorexia nervosa: Pragmatic randomised controlled trial. *BJPsych Open, 20*, 56–66.

Hooley, J. M., & Richters, J. E. (1995). Expressed emotion: A developmental perspective. In D. Cicchetti & S. L. Toth (Eds.), *Rochester symposium on developmental psychopathology, Vol. 6: Emotion, cognition, and representation* (pp. 133–166). Rochester, NY: University of Rochester Press.

King, S. (2000). Is expressed emotion cause or effect in the mothers of schizophrenic young adults? *Schizophrenia Research, 45*, 65–78.

Leff, J. (1989). Controversial issues and growing points in research on relatives' expressed emotion. *The International Journal of Social Psychiatry, 35*, 133–145.

Leff, J., & Vaughn, C. (1985). *Expressed emotion in families: Its significance for mental illness.* New York: Guilford Press.

Liakopoulou, M., Alifieraki, T., Katideniou, A., Peppa, M., Maniati, M., Tzikas, D., . . . Dacou-Voutetakis, C. (2001). Maternal expressed emotion and metabolic control of children and adolescents with diabetes mellitus. *Psychotherapy and Psychosomatics, 70*, 78–85.

Öksüz, E., Karaca, S., Özaltin, G., & Ateş, M. A. (2017). The effects of psychoeducation on the expressed emotion and family functioning of the family members in first-episode schizophrenia. *Community Mental Health Journal, 53*, 464–473.

Rienecke, R. D. (2018). Expressed emotion and eating disorders: An updated review. *Current Psychiatry Reviews, 14*, 84–98.

Rutter, M., & Brown, G. W. (1966). The reliability and validity of measures of family life and relationships in families containing a psychiatric patient. *Social Psychiatry, 1*, 38–53.

Uehara, T., Kawashima, Y., Goto, M., Tasaki, S., & Someya, T. (2001). Psychoeducation for the families of patients with eating disorders and changes in expressed emotion: A preliminary study. *Comprehensive Psychiatry, 42*, 132–138.

Uehara, T., Yokoyama, T., Goto, M., & Ihda, S. (1996). Expressed emotion and short-term treatment outcome of outpatients with major depression. *Comprehensive Psychiatry, 37*, 299–304.

Vaughn, C. E., & Leff, J. P. (1976a). The measurement of expressed emotion in the families of psychiatric patients. *British Journal of Social and Clinical Psychology, 15*, 157–165.

Vaughn, C. E., & Leff, J. P. (1976b). The influence of family and social factors on the course of psychiatric illness: A comparison of schizophrenic and depressed neurotic patients. *British Journal of Psychiatry*, *129*, 125–137.

Wearden, A. J., Tarrier, N., Barrowclough, C., Zastowny, T. R., & Rahill, A. A. (2000). A review of expressed emotion research in health care. *Clinical Psychology Review*, *20*, 633–666.

Whitney, J., & Eisler, I. (2005). Theoretical and empirical models around caring for someone with an eating disorder: The reorganization of family life and inter-personal maintenance factors. *Journal of Mental Health*, *14*, 575–585.

2

Expressed Emotion and Psychosis

Juliana Onwumere and Elizabeth Kuipers

Background

Schizophrenia spectrum disorders (e.g. schizophrenia, schizoaffective disorder), which are commonly and collectively referred to as psychosis, are severe mental health conditions affecting several million people across the world. Recent data reported pooled incidence rates of psychotic disorders were 26.6 per 100 000 person-years (95% confidence interval 22.0–31.7) with elevated rates in minority ethnic groups and in males (Jongsma, Turner, Kirkbride, & Jones, 2019). Schizophrenia is ranked, globally, in the top 15 disorders leading to disability (Charlson et al., 2018). The first episode of psychosis typically emerges during late adolescence and young adulthood, a period of significant developmental, emotional and social transition. The defining symptoms often include hallucinations in different sensory modalities (e.g. auditory verbal hallucinations), delusions, and thought disorder alongside marked disturbances in mood, cognition, social and vocational functioning (Fleischhacker et al., 2014; Velthorst et al., 2016). For many of those affected, psychosis disorders are experienced as a long-term and socially disabling condition. The conditions generally have a relapsing and remitting course with elevated levels of relapse within the first two to five years following onset (Robinson et al., 1999; Zipursky, Menezes, & Streiner, 2014; Pelayo-Terán et al., 2017).

When compared with the general population, adults living with psychosis disorders have a reduced life expectancy of approximately 15–20 years (Hayes et al., 2017). In addition, there are elevated rates of social isolation, childhood victimization, and trauma in those diagnosed with the condition (Gayer-Anderson & Morgan, 2013; Sündermann et al., 2014).

Psychosis and Family Support

Although people with psychosis have small social networks, many have contact with informal carers, typically close relatives such as parents, partners, siblings, and adult children (Palumbo, Volpe, Matanov, Priebe, & Giacco, 2015). These relatives have assumed a caregiving role with little preparation or choice and do the bulk of their learning on the job and through trial and error. An increasing body of research evidence and clinical experience underscores the relevance and importance of carer support to improving service user outcomes in psychosis. The estimated financial cost of informal caregiver support for people with psychosis exceeds 1.2 billion U.K. pounds per annum (The Schizophrenia Commission, 2012), with similar figures reported in other regions of the world. We know that carer support remains a key component in an individual's ability to access appropriate care at first episode (Jansen, Gleeson, & Cotton, 2015; Fridgen et al., 2013). It also has an influential role in significantly decreasing levels of psychosis relapse and hospitalization (Norman et al., 2005), improving levels of patient engagement in treatments (Lucksted et al., 2018), and improving mortality rates (Revier et al., 2015). In a 14-year follow up of patients with psychosis living in China, an absence of family support was associated with greater rates of homelessness and mortality (Ran et al., 2016).

Impact of Care

Similar to patterns observed in other health problems, psychosis not only affects the person with the diagnosis but also those in their networks. The impact of the caregiving role on carer health and wellbeing outcomes has been well documented with an acknowledgment that caregiving experiences in psychosis are multifaceted. Thus, as part of their role, carers have reported a broad range of positive experiences and outcomes that have included enhanced self-esteem and self-confidence; improved knowledge; understanding, empathy, and compassion about and towards people with mental health disabilities and their challenges; and improved quality of their relationship with the person they care for and family solidarity (Chen & Greenberg, 2004; Hsiao & Tsai, 2014; Shiraishi & Reilly, 2019). Positive caregiving experiences are independent of negative experiences. Thus, they can exist in parallel with or positioned within negative aspects (Onwumere et al., 2008; Shiraishi & Reilly, 2019) but with their own underlying factors (Jansen et al., 2015). To date, however, much greater attention has been given to the less positive and the problematic aspects of the psychosis caregiving role, including the experience of burden and difficult family relationships.

In carers, per se, irrespective of the specific health condition affecting their relative, data from general population health surveys confirm a greater proportion of common mental disorders in carers versus non-carer peers. The positive link between caregiving status and higher levels of mental health disorders were evident for those engaged in ten hours a week of caregiving or greater and with a twofold increase in those engaged in care at 20 hours or more each week (Smith et al., 2014). Legg et al. (2012) offered similar observations of poor health status in 5,451,902 informal carers compared with the general population and greater difficulties with more caregiving hours, particularly for those engaged in caregiving for 20 hours or more a week.

When we consider carers for people with psychosis, specifically, there are elevated rates of low mood and stress related conditions, including burnout (Gupta, Isherwood, Jones, & Van Impe, 2015; Kuipers, Onwumere, & Bebbington, 2010; Onwumere et al., 2017; Sadath, Muralidhar, Varambally, Gangadhar, & Rose, 2017). It is estimated that between 30% and 40% of carers in psychosis experience clinical depression and psychological distress (Hamaie et al., 2016; Hayes, Hawthorne, Farhall, O'Hanlon, & Harvey, 2015), while reports of distress are particularly elevated during the first episode (Sadath et al., 2017; Jansen et al., 2015; MCann, Lubman, & Clark, 2011). Trauma symptoms are recorded in approximately 40% of carers (Kingston, Onwumere, Keen, Ruffell, & Kuipers, 2016; Barton & Jackson, 2008). Carers encounter a broad range of patient behaviors that can be unusual in presentation and difficult to make sense of and deal with. This can also involve behaviors that leave carers feeling hurt and concerned about their safety (Onwumere et al., 2014; Onwumere, Zhou, & Kuipers, 2018; Smith et al, 2018). Approximately one third of carers have been the victim of patient violence during the preceding 12 months (Kageyama et al., 2016). Data comparison of families of parental carers of people with schizophrenia, rheumatoid arthritis, multiple sclerosis, or epilepsy with healthy control participants found significantly higher risk in carers of people with schizophrenia for their use of psychiatric healthcare. Moreover, their use of services tended to progress over time in tandem with poorer patient health (Mittendorfer-Rutz et al., 2019). Pan-European survey data confirm high levels of isolation and poor social networks in carers, which exceed levels observed in similar burdensome health conditions (e.g. stroke, brain injury) (Magliano, Fiorillo, De Rosa, Malangone, Maj, & National Mental Health Working Group, 2005).

The physical health outcomes of carers are also impacted by the caregiving role (Perlick et al., 2005). Pain and an overall poorer level of health-related quality of life are observed in carers (Gupta et al., 2015). These types of problems are already observable during the early course of the mental health difficulties. Sleep difficulties, as measured by the Pittsburgh Sleep Quality Index (Buysse et al., 1989), have been reported in approximately two thirds of early psychosis carers (Smith et al., 2018). Poon, Curtis, Ward, Lonergan, and Lappin (2018) reported that at first-episode psychosis, approximately 40% of carers present as being at high risk for type 2 diabetes, 80% are overweight, and one third have hypertension.

Expressed Emotion in Caregiving Relationships in Psychosis

As reported in the opening chapters, expressed emotion (EE) attitudes and behaviors map onto five domains (Critical Comments, Hostility, Emotional Overinvolvement [EOI], Warmth, and Positive Remarks). A high EE rating reflects above threshold levels of Criticism and/orHostility and/or EOI towards the person they care for (Vaughn & Leff, 1976). Low EE ratings reflect carers who did not score above threshold on any of these three scales. EE ratings offer a quantifiable marker of family atmosphere and are a strong predictor of *patient outcomes*. Across many groups in psychosis (but not all), high EE ratings are linked to significantly higher rates of patient relapse and hospitalization (Weintraub et al., 2017), longer hospital admissions (Marom, Munitz, Jones, Weizman, & Hermesh, 2005), and a shorter time to relapse (Koutra et al., 2015). Data from the first review and aggregate analysis of EE studies in psychosis confirmed that in high-EE caregiving relationships, patients experienced relapse rates at least twice the level as peers from low-EE relationships (Bebbington & Kuipers, 1994). These findings were later supported by similar work from Butzlaff and Hooley (1998). Data from a recent meta analyses of 34 EE outcome studies ($k = 34$, $N = 1{,}982$) indicated that high EE (versus low EE) provided a 95% increased likelihood of relapse (O'Driscoll, Sener, Angmark, & Shaikh, 2019). Over time, further evidence has highlighted the importance of criticism within EE and its strength for predicting greater levels of patient relapse and poorer patient outcomes at the first episode stage and beyond (Alvarez-Jimenez et al., 2012). Cechnicki, Bielanska, Hanuszkiewicz, and Daren (2013) examined 43 adults with psychosis over 20 years (i.e. year 1, 3, 7, 12, 20) and identified significantly higher relapse rates at all time points from year 3 to 20 in high-EE groups. Greater relapse levels were associated with higher levels of Critical Comments. Criticism is also linked to poor patient outcomes, including greater cannabis use (Gonzalez-Blanch et al., 2015) and greater patient paranoia at 12-month follow ups (Hesse et al., 2015).

Patients in high-EE caregiving relationships are also more likely to report mood disturbances in terms of greater anxiety and anger and lower mood and self-esteem (Finnegan et al., 2014; Docherty et al., 2011; Barrowclough et al., 2003) and to engage in more physical violence towards their carers (Kageyama & Solomon, 2018). Recent evidence from a study of adults with low risk versus elevated risk of developing schizophrenia showed no differences in their subjective mood and physiological reactions immediately following their exposure to carer criticism. However, in the elevated-risk group, there was evidence of significantly higher physiological disturbance, in terms of greater heart activation, during the recovery period. In other words, individuals at elevated risk for developing psychosis appeared to have greater sensitivity in dealing with or recovering from the effects of criticism (Weintraub et al., 2018). Interestingly, differential patterns of brain functioning have also been recorded in patients following their exposure to low- and high-EE communications from carers. High-EE communications are linked to activation in brain regions responsible for the processing of aversive social information (e.g. rostral anterior cingulate, middle superior frontal gyrus) (Rylands et al., 2010).

As mentioned previously, established and predictive links between high-EE and poorer patient outcomes are recorded in patient caregiver groups in psychosis (Bebbington & Kuipers, 1994; Weintraub, Hall, Carbonella, Weisman De Manani, & Hooley, 2017) but not uniformly so (Bhugra & McKenzie, 2003). For example, in some studies using African American samples, low-EE caregiving relationships have been associated with greater patient symptomatology (Gurak & Weisman de Mamani, 2017), and high-EE relationships, in the form of criticism and EOI, were predictive of improved patient outcomes compared with non-Hispanic white American peers when the traditional EE poor patient outcomes were observed (Rosenfarb et al., 2006). Similarly, EE data from Mexican and Latin American groups found that negative patient outcomes, including relapse, were not predicted by high EE but by the absence of prosocial aspects within a caregiving relationship (i.e. warmth) (López et al., 2004).

EE, Illness Beliefs, and Coping

EE relationships, particularly those rated as high EE, offer clinically important information that extends beyond their predictive links with poorer patient outcomes. Thus, they can often provide a framework for a more detailed understanding of the appraisals carers report about the illness and of themselves such as attributions of blame about illness cause and beliefs about illness length and perceived consequences (e.g. Dominguez-Marinez, Medina-Pradas, Kwapil, & Barrantes-Vidal, 2017; Kuipers et al., 2007). For example, high-EE relationships that are characterized by criticism and hostility are positively linked with "responsibility attributions". These are beliefs that their relative is to blame for their difficulties and could stop such difficulties if they chose to (Barrowclough & Hooley, 2003). In a study of 35 relatives of adults with psychosis and 42 relatives of adults with depression, high-EE carers (versus low EE groups) were found to attribute greater control to patients but also to behave in a more controlling manner towards their relatives (Hooley & Campbell, 2002). Cherry et al. (2018) reported that carers high on criticism and hostility were more likely to have avoidant attachment styles and less abilities to mentalize and therefore make sense of their own actions, thoughts, and feelings and those of others. In contrast, high-EE relationships due to EOI behaviors are predominately linked to carer beliefs of self-blame and guilt. These are carers who hold themselves responsible for their relative's mental health problems and perceive their relative as having little or no control over their difficulties (Barrowclough & Hooley, 2003). More recent work from Cherry and colleagues (2017) extend these findings to suggest that carers with EOI are also more inclined to experience feelings of shame. Carers experiencing higher levels of burden and psychological distress are also more likely to engage in avoidant and less effective coping strategies (Onwumere et al., 2011). Further, these carers are more likely to be recorded as being in high-EE relationships (Jansen et al., 2014).

EE and Patient Appraisals

Empirical evidence indicates that people living with psychosis have a greater sensitivity towards affective attitudes and behaviors from others and can accurately perceive negative affect from caregivers (Onwumere et al., 2009; Weintraub et al., 2018). Patient perceptions of carer behaviors and affect can also impact their own functioning and wellbeing (Tomlinson, Onwumere, & Kuipers, 2014), and the impact can be more important than effects of carer-reported EE on patient outcomes (Tompson et al., 1995).

Positive Family Relationships

Since the very early studies of EE (Brown et al., 1962), the important contribution of warmth and positive family environments in optimizing patient outcomes in psychosis has been highlighted, albeit with less research focus (Butler, Berry, Ellet, & Bucci, 2019). The predictive links between high EE and poorer patient outcomes (e.g. greater relapse rates) has, unfortunately, eclipsed research efforts and clinical approaches about the broader contribution of EE ratings.

Nevertheless, carer warmth has been linked with reduced relapse rates (Bertrando et al., 1992; Bebbington & Kuipers, 1994), including for those at first episode (Lee, Barrowclough, & Lobban, 2014) and specifically amongst some cultural groups (e.g. Mexican American) (Breitborde, López, Wickens, Jenkins, & Karno, 2007). In patients experiencing first-episode psychosis, significantly lower rates of relapse at 6 months and 12 months of follow up were recorded when carers were rated highly for warmth or when patients perceived more positive affect from carers (Lee et al., 2014). In at-risk psychosis groups, carer warmth has been predictive of increased social functioning (O'Brien et al., 2006, 2008; Schlosser et al., 2010). Interestingly, Butler et al. (2019) completed an analogue study in a non-clinical sample and confirmed the positive relationship between criticism exposure and paranoia. However, the addition of warmth was insufficient by itself to significantly reduce the effects of the criticism.

Working With Families in Psychosis: The Contribution of EE

The importance of EE to patient outcomes was one of the initial drivers of the original development of cognitive behavioral–based family interventions for psychosis (e.g Kuipers, Leff, & Lam, 2002; Barrowclough & Tarrier, 1992; Falloon, Boyd, & McGill, 1984). Family interventions in psychosis (FIp) are evidence-based psychological talking therapies that involve working with patients and carers together or carers alone and are recommended treatments in many areas across the globe, including Europe, Canada, Australia, and the US (Galletly et al., 2016; Norman, Buchanan, Dickerson, & Dixon, 2017; Kreyenbuhl, Buchanan, Dickerson, & Dixon, 2010; S3 guidelines), as well as in the U.K. (National Institute for Heath and Care Excellence; NICE, 2014).

Some of the goals in family interventions are to reduce levels of Criticism, Hostility, and EOI in high-EE families but also to increase positive interactions and warmth (Kuipers et al., 2002). These changes are achieved via key methods, which include psychoeducation, skills facilitation in problem solving, adaptive coping, and positive communication, as well as cognitive reappraisal and positive reframing. FIp implementation in service settings can be low (Ince, Haddock, & Tai, 2016) despite the robust and expanding evidence base (Pharoah, Mari, Rathbone, & Wong, 2010; Claxton, Onwumere, & Fornells-Ambrojo, 2017; Camacho-Gomez & Castellvi, 2019) and treatment guidelines and recommendations (NICE, 2014). Poor provision of such treatments has been attributed to several factors, including difficulties of engaging patients and carers together (Onwumere, Grice, & Kuipers, 2016).

Interestingly, interventions to support patients to cope with perceived negative family interactions have received limited attention in the literature, despite the evidence of the direct effects of criticism on patients (Finnegan et al., 2014). There is limited literature on individual psychological interventions designed specifically for people with psychosis reporting interpersonal difficulties with a carer. It is possible, however, that modified components of FIp that have also supported work with high-EE caregiving relationships could be applied directly with individual patients. Cognitive reappraisal and reframing are aspects of FIp that could support patients to deal with the emotional impact of negative caregiving relationships (e.g. perceived criticism [PC] from carers). These interventions can be supported by strategies to enhance self-esteem and techniques (e.g. role-play, rehearsal) to embed learning.

Cognitive Reappraisal

Cognitive distortions play a key role in the ontogeny and maintenance of emotional dysfunction in adults, through processes such as overgeneralization and selective attention. Cognitive reappraisal is defined as changing the meaning individuals assign to a situation and by doing so, altering its emotional impact (Gross, 2002). Individuals who utilize reappraisal can experience less negative emotion (Gross, 2001) and better self-reported interpersonal functioning (Gross & John, 2003).

Cognitive Reframing

Cognitive reframing is a therapeutic skill used in family treatments. It can be helpful in managing negative communications between family members and ensuring underlying emotional issues (e.g. concern) are identified.

Enhancing Self-Esteem

Negative self-concept features in many mental health conditions, including psychosis (Smith et al., 2006), and serves as a vulnerability factor for relapse (Garety, Kuipers, Fowler, Freeman, & Bebbington, 2001). In psychosis, reports of carer criticism are associated with patients' negative self-appraisal (Kuipers et al., 2006). Further, patient perceptions of negative family interactions are predictive of negative self-concepts and poorer symptom functioning (Hesse et al., 2015). Hall and Tarrier (2003) developed a brief and effective cognitive-behavioral therapy (CBT)–informed intervention designed to enhance self-esteem in people with psychosis. The main focus centered on encouraging patients to elicit statements about their positive qualities, identifying evidence to support these statements over the following week, and monitoring belief change.

Role-Play and Rehearsal

Role-play is a teaching strategy employed to promote active learning (Van Ments, 1999) and is defined as an experiment in which the person is asked to behave *as if* they were an individual in a given situation (Aronson & Carlsmith, 1968). In family work, role-play offers an important tool in helping individuals to gain the perspective of another and to develop confidence in implementing new skills.

Case Descriptions: Targeting Negative Emotional Sequelae of Perceived Expressed in Patients With Psychosis

In the next part of this chapter, we outline three case descriptions of the initial application of a novel therapeutic approach, incorporating key FIp techniques of cognitive reappraisal and positive reframing, combined with self-esteem enhancement and role-play. The novel approach was designed to reduce the negative impact on patients with psychosis of perceived negative EE communications from carers. The intervention was led by doctoral-level, clinical psychologist in training (Finnegan, 2011). All personal identifiable details have been altered. Participants were eligible for inclusion if they were aged 18–65 years, with a case note diagnosis of schizophrenia spectrum, and had a caregiver who they perceived as critical of them and were not currently receiving psychological therapy. After consent, participants attended three individual sessions with the therapist starting with (1) a baseline assessment session (45 minutes), (2) an intervention session (90 minutes), and (3) a follow-up meeting after one week (60 minutes). Ethical approval for the study, including informed and written consent for publication from participants, was provided by the North London Ethical Committee (10/HO717/72).

Intervention Approach

Session 1

Participants were asked about perceived negative communication with carers that were recorded in a diary (a basic version of a thought diary used in traditional CBT). The diary recorded negative automatic thoughts (NATs), negative communication, and the degree to which these were linked to negative affect. A meeting was set up for one week later.

Session 2

Participants were asked to identify one example of a recent perceived negative interaction between their carer and themselves associated with negative affect, which was then used to introduce cognitive reappraisal and reframing strategies. *Reappraising* negative communication involved a focus on cognitively restructuring the participant's view of (1) the negative interaction and (2) the carer. The aim was to help participants adopt a less negative and self-blaming view. *Reframing* negative communication involved exploring how it was neither synonymous with nor confirmation of a negative perception of the patient and their worth. Exploration of potential issues that underpinned comments (e.g. carer concern) was also reviewed. In session, the reappraisal and reframe was entered in the negative communication diary. The participant was then encouraged to identify another typical example to use as role-play. The therapist played the carer and the participant themselves. Participants were asked to verbally rehearse the reappraisal and reframing techniques. Another diary entry was completed with the participant's reappraisal and reframe recorded.

At the end of session 2, participants were asked to keep a positive qualities journal for one week. Participants recorded what their carer would describe as being the participant's most positive quality and their carer's most positive quality plus evidence of these qualities and a rating of how strongly they believed them on a scale of 0–100. This was done to increase participants' positive sense of self (self-esteem) and encourage more positive relationships.

Session 3 – One-Week Follow Up

A week after session 2, in the third and final session, participants reflected upon the therapy process and provided feedback.

Case 1 – Mike

BACKGROUND

Mike was in his late 20s, diagnosed with schizoaffective disorder six years previously, and lived with his parents. His main psychosis symptoms included paranoid beliefs and auditory hallucinations. He was under the care of a community mental health team (CMHT) and had recently commenced voluntary work two days per week and was planning to re-start his education.

NEGATIVE COMMUNICATIONS

- Financial contribution to household: Mike's parents often said: "Haven't you found a job yet?" He felt that their questions meant they did not "respect" his decision to attend college and that his father would prefer him to contribute financially.
- Household rules: negative communications about Mike's uncompleted household chores and use of the bathroom.
- Perceived invalidation of illness: parents often made comments such as "You're fine now – you're recovered". Mike felt that his struggles, including residual positive symptoms of psychosis, were not understood.

PATHWAY BETWEEN NEGATIVE COMMUNICATION AND SYMPTOMS OF PSYCHOSIS

Through completing the negative communication diaries, a formulation was developed about the effect of Mike's reports of criticism from his parents. Using a recent example, when he told his mother about starting voluntary work, he perceived her response as critical. The NATs were "I'm not good enough" (90%) and "My illness is not taken seriously" (90%). These thoughts elicited a core belief "I'm a loser" (100%). Supporting evidence was that his parents "constantly ask me if I have a job" and often "undermine my illness". These thoughts left him feeling sad (70%) and angry (80%) and precipitated a cycle of arguments, anger, withdrawing to his bedroom, and a worsening of his anxiety and paranoia.

NEGATIVE COMMUNICATION DIARIES

During session 2, Mike's example of PC was used to elicit evidence *against* his NATs. Mike acknowledged that although this is what he inferred and concluded, his mother had never actually told him that she thought he was "lazy" even during arguments. She had also seemed sympathetic when he had mentioned experiencing unwanted side effects from his medication.

REAPPRAISING

This involved examining Mike's thinking style and generating more positive alternatives. Mike thought that his parents did not take his psychosis and ongoing symptoms seriously. A more positive appraisal was that his diagnosis was upsetting for his parents, which would account for their questioning. He also wondered whether his own reasoning was too emotional. He acknowledged that just because it *felt* like his parents did not take his illness seriously did not mean it was true.

REFRAMING

Reframing involved exploring how Mike's perception of parental criticism may also be his parents' way of expressing concern. In the example of his parents' inquiry about job opportunities, Mike and the therapist considered how his parents might view his current situation and what their concerns might be. Mike wondered whether his mother was worried about his recovery and had worries of her own about whether they were doing enough or had "failed him". The perceived Critical Comments from his parents about employment were reframed as their way of expressing worry and concern for him because they were worried about how he might survive when they were no longer around to offer support.

ROLE-PLAYING

Following the reappraising and reframing discussions, Mike role-played a typical verbal exchange with his father that focused on "household rules" (the shower rota). The therapist assumed the role of Mike's father, and Mike played himself. There was a discussion over whether the rules were in place to minimize conflict and any negative effect on Mike and the wider family. The final part of the discussion focused on whether Mike was, understandably, hypervigilant about perceived negative comments, which, in turn, sometimes meant he was perhaps too ready to take the content of discussions with his parents as evidence that they did not care about him. When Mike reframed and reappraised his example of negative communication using negative communication diaries, taking the evidence against his NATs into account, he modified the emotions that he felt. He reported that he would feel less sad (60%, a decrease of 10%) and angry (65%, a decrease of 15%).

POSITIVE QUALITIES JOURNAL

Mike and the therapist completed one example of the positive qualities journal in the session. For the following week, Mike recorded what his mother would describe as his positive qualities and what he considered as his mother's positive qualities. This included what they liked about one another, what their biggest achievements were, the challenges they had faced in their lives, their talents, their good values. Mike provided examples of communication during the week that demonstrated some of these positive qualities. He also rated how strongly he believed them to be accurate on a scale of 0–100.

FEEDBACK, SESSION 3, ONE-WEEK FOLLOW UP

Mike reported feeling more sympathetic toward his parents. He felt he had been able to communicate with his parents about household issues and vocational plans, without experiencing the typical negative emotional sequelae. Mike's mother had acknowledged that she often worried about him and did not always cope well. Mike felt able to share his positive qualities journal with his mother and that she had given him positive feedback about himself to record in the journal. Mike reported that talking about the situations that elicited negative communication between him and his parents had felt challenging but worthwhile.

Case 2 – Daniel

BACKGROUND

Daniel, in his early 30s, had an approximate 11-year history of schizoaffective disorder. His main symptoms included delusional beliefs, auditory hallucinations, and social functioning difficulties. He had five or six previous hospital admissions, and he was under the care of a CMHT. Daniel was attending a college course and living at home with his mother.

NEGATIVE COMMUNICATIONS

- Lifestyle habits and physical health: Daniel reported having regular disagreements with his mother about his health and lifestyle choices (e.g. smoking) and their impact on his health.
- Financial: Daniel reported disagreements and negative exchanges with his mother about money and payment for household bills.

PATHWAY BETWEEN NEGATIVE COMMUNICATION AND SYMPTOMS OF PSYCHOSIS

Daniel linked the perceived negative interaction with his mother to difficulties with his mood, which in turn had a negative impact on his psychosis experiences, particularly levels of paranoid thinking. Daniel reported that he had recently had a difficult exchange with his mother over what was considered his lack of willingness to complete a household chore. He reported that his mother had accused him of not doing enough around the house, and the comments left him feeling upset (80%) and scared (80%). He listed his NATs as "I am a disappointment to my mother" (90%) and "I am useless" (90%). These thoughts were linked to a core belief "I am bad" (100%). The supporting evidence for these thoughts was the fact that he did not "have a job or a child", both of which he felt were expected of a man of his age and background.

NEGATIVE COMMUNICATION DIARIES

During session 2, the therapist used Daniel's example of a recent negative communication (i.e. sorting items for laundry) to elicit evidence *against* his NATs. Daniel acknowledged that his mother often praised him when he helped around the house. He also reported that she had told him that she was proud of how he was managing his studies.

REAPPRAISING

Reappraising his mother's perceived Critical Comments involved exploring Daniel's thinking style around their arguments and generating more positive interpretations (i.e less blaming) and alternative meanings for the comments. Daniel reappraised his baseline view that his mother was "a very angry woman" who only wanted to upset him. Instead, she was reappraised as a strong, outspoken woman, qualities he had always valued.

He recounted how his mother had stood by him throughout his problems and how her strong will ensured that he received the help that he needed. He noted that his mother had little support and probably found it difficult to cope at times. He wondered whether this impacted on how felt and communicated with him.

REFRAMING

Daniel spoke about feeling criticized by his mother for not being employed and linked this to not having his own family. The therapist thought about how his mother might view the situation and what her concerns might be. Daniel reported that his mother was a migrant to the country and thought the most important achievements in life for any man were to have a wife and children of his own and to support his family financially. He thought that his mother was probably concerned about him not achieving these goals, because "she loves me and would like me to be happy".

ROLE-PLAYING

In the role-play exercise, Daniel used an example of his mother telling him not to smoke in their house. He felt able to discuss with his mother the reasons he wanted to smoke but in a less emotionally charged way. When Daniel reframed and reappraised his example of negative communication using the negative communication diaries, taking the evidence against his NATs into account, he modified the emotions that he felt. He reported that he would only feel 2% sad (a decrease of 78%) and 2% scared (a decrease of 78%).

POSITIVE QUALITIES JOURNAL

Daniel and the therapist used part of the session to document endearing and positive qualities his mother would use to describe him and qualities he perceived as positive in her.

FEEDBACK, SESSION 3, ONE-WEEK FOLLOW UP

Daniel reported appraising the disagreements with his mother in a more positive way following the intervention. He still had incidents of PC during the week but felt they were both "very similar people" and he could understand her perspective more. He stated that he could see how much his mother loved and cared for him, and that their arguments were "just her way of coping with difficult situations".

Case 3 – Sam

BACKGROUND

Sam was a man in his early 20s who had been diagnosed with paranoid schizophrenia six years previously. Sam was working as a special needs assistant. He lived at home with his parents and described his mother as his main carer.

NEGATIVE COMMUNICATIONS

- Intrusion: Sam reported that his mother often "butts into my business". He felt that his mother "treats me like a child". He reported that his mother often spoke to his key worker about his symptoms and treatment, gave unnecessary reminders, and ignored the fact that he was an adult with a job.

PATHWAY BETWEEN NEGATIVE COMMUNICATION AND SYMPTOMS OF PSYCHOSIS

Sam reported that although he was not currently experiencing problematic symptoms like he had in the past, he worried that if he continued to experience negative communication with his mother, he would become unwell again. Sam explained that he and his mother often disagreed when he was driving, or he failed to follow her unsolicited advice on how he should drive. This left him feeling irritated (65%) and sad (70%). His NATs were "I can never do anything right" (90%) and "This is unfair – she treats me like I'm a child" (90%). He reported that these thoughts elicited a core belief "I am incompetent" (80%). He took his mother's need to tell him what to do "all the time" as supporting evidence for his own incompetence and had begun to feel it was gradually "wearing me down".

NEGATIVE COMMUNICATION DIARIES

During session 2, the therapist used Sam's example (his mother commenting on his driving) to elicit evidence *against* his NATs. Sam acknowledged that there were certain areas of his life that were not a source of arguments between his mother and himself.

REAPPRAISING

Reappraising the perceived Critical Comments from his mother involved considering potential reasons underpinning his mother's behavior and any concerns that she might have had. Sam reported that previously, his mother had told him that she "felt responsible" for his psychiatric problems. He questioned whether she was always blaming herself and feeling guilty, which might affect how she behaved towards him.

REFRAMING

Sam spoke about feeling incompetent as his mother often interfered and took over. He acknowledged that, regarding his driving, his mother wanted him (and herself) to be safe because of love and concern. Similarly, he linked his mother's reminders about his treatment to underlying love, concern and anxiety about him.

ROLE-PLAYING

Following the reappraising and reframing, Sam was encouraged to role-play a typical argument with his mother. The scenario was a situation when Sam became aware that his mother was commenting on his medication with his primary care physician and arguing with her about this and clarifying how it made him feel.

When Sam reframed and reappraised the negative communication, taking the evidence against his NATs into account, he was able to modify the emotions that he felt such that he reported he would feel 50% sad (a decrease of 20%).

POSITIVE QUALITIES JOURNAL

The same procedure employed with Mike and Daniel was used in the case of Sam.

FEEDBACK, SESSION 3, ONE-WEEK FOLLOW UP

Sam reported feeling greater empathy for his mother following the session. He continued to find her behavior bothersome, but less so, and felt equipped to discuss his driving without it automatically leading to an argument.

Case Reflection

These case descriptions describe the initial application of a brief psychological intervention designed to support individuals with psychosis to deal with effects of perceived negative EE communications. The intervention incorporates components of evidence-based FIp alongside self-esteem–enhancing approaches and role-play. Although the intervention appeared acceptable, we note that without a controlled design and objective and quantitative measures, it is not possible to reliably attribute subjectively reported changes to the intervention. We also acknowledge that non-specific therapy-related factors (e.g. therapist contact) were likely to have impacted the patient experience. That said, preliminary feedback offers modest indications of its possible potential value and a pathway for further research on working with patient experiences and perceptions of carer EE. We already know that individuals who are emotionally affected by perceptions of carer criticism and who do not utilize reappraisal and reframing strategies may be particularly vulnerable to negative outcomes (Onwumere et al., 2009). If these individuals could be targeted, this might be one way for improving outcomes while maintaining the supportive aspects of having a social network.

All participants commented on challenges the interventions presented such as generating counter evidence, using role-play, which they were unfamiliar with and remembering to complete the journal during the week. The latter is common in CBT psychosis-based interventions, and cognitive problems (e.g. working memory difficulties) are highly prevalent in psychosis (Wood, Cupitt, & Lavender, 2015). For future iterations of this approach, these issues must be considered. The sessions were closely supervised by an expert clinician in individual and family-based CBT interventions in psychosis. As noted by Roth and Pilling (2013), it would not be recommended to carry out this type of interventions without adequate supervision.

Many individuals living with psychosis will not engage with evidence-based family interventions despite having poor relationships, which may impede their recovery and day-to-day wellbeing. This kind of direct intervention may have potential and be more feasible.

Conclusion

Research on the effects of difficult relationships on both carers and people with psychosis is now well established as leading to poorer outcomes. While family interventions are recommended for those with family members with psychosis, as is support for carers, implementation of these interventions has been problematic. Most families still do not receive this kind of help, although first-episode teams are more likely to do this now than has been the case in the past. An alternative approach might be to offer help directly to patients with psychosis who report difficult, including critical, relationships with close family members. Some examples of how this could be done using a range of standard techniques from the family intervention in psychosis literature have been presented. Flexible, direct approaches with patients on their own may have particular clinical value when family sessions are not possible or appropriate and may offer another way of dealing with negative interactions. The effectiveness of such approaches has yet to be demonstrated, but the case studies presented suggest that these kinds of individual interventions may be feasible and extend the clinical utility of EE. Although the EE concept remains relevant and measurable in diverse cultural groups, the predictive links of high EE and poorer outcomes are not uniform. As we move forward with EE research, there remains a clear clinical need and rationale for further inquiry that explores EE within a cultural framework and considers its implications for supporting families.

References

Alvarez-Jimenez, M., Priede, A., Hetrick, S. E., Bendall, S., Killackey, E., Parker, A. G., McGorry, P. D., & Gleeson, J. F. (2012). Risk actors for relapse following treatment for first episode psychosis: a systematic review and meta-analysis of longitudinal studies. *Schizophrenia Research*, *139*, 116–128.

Aronson, E., & Carlsmith, J. M. (1968). Experimentation in social psychology. In G. Lindzey & E. Aronson (Eds.), *Handbook of social psychology* (3rd ed., pp. 441–486). Reading, UK: Addison-Wesley.

Barrowclough, C., & Hooley, J. M. (2003). Attributions and expressed emotion: A review. *Clinical Psychology Review*, *23*, 849–880.

Barrowclough, C., & Tarrier, N. (1992). *Families of schizophrenic patients: Cognitive behavioural interventions*. Cheltenham, UK: Nelson Thornes.

Barrowclough, C., Tarrier, N., Humphreys, L., Ward, J., Gregg, L., & Andrews, B. (2003). Self-esteem in schizophrenia: Relationships between self-evaluation, family attitudes, and symptomatology. *Journal of Abnormal Psychology*, *112*(1), 92–99.

Barton, K., & Jackson, C. (2008). Reducing symptoms of trauma among carers of people with psychosis: Pilot study examining the impact of writing about caregiving experiences. *Australian and New Zealand Journal of Psychiatry, 42*, 693–701. doi:10.1080/00048670802203434

Bebbington, P., & Kuipers, L. (1994). The predictive utility of expressed emotion in schizophrenia: An aggregate analysis. *Psychological Medicine, 24*(3), 707–718.

Bertrando, P., Beltz, J., Bressi, C., Clerici, M., Farma, T., Invernizzi, G., & Cazzullo, C. L. (1992). Expressed emotion and schizophrenia in Italy: A study of an urban population. *British Journal of Psychiatry, 161*, 223–229.

Bhugra, D., & McKenzie, K. (2003). Expressed emotion across cultures. *Advances in Psychiatric Treatment, 9*(5), 342–348.

Breitborde, N. J., López, S. R., Wickens, T. D., Jenkins, J. H., & Karno, M. (2007). Toward specifying the nature of the relationship between expressed emotion and schizophrenic relapse: The utility of curvilinear models. *International Journal of Methods of Psychiatric Research, 16*(1), 1–10.

Brown, G. W., Monck, E. M., Carstairs, G. M., & Wing, J. K. (1962). Influence of family life on the course of schizophrenic illness. *British Journal of Preventive & Social Medicine, 16*, 55–68.

Butler, R., Berry, K., Ellet, L., & Bucci, S. (2019). An experimental investigation of the impact of critical and warm comments on state paranoia in a non-clinical sample. *Journal of Behaviour Therapy and Experimental Psychiatry, 62*, 30–37.

Butzlaff, R. L., & Hooley, J. M. (1988). Expressed emotion and psychiatric relapse: A meta-analysis. *Archives of General Psychiatry, 55*, 547–552.

Buysse, D. J., Reynolds III, C. F., Monk, T. H., Berman, S. R., & Kupfer, D. J. (1989). The Pittsburgh Sleep Quality Index: A new instrument for psychiatric practice and research. *Psychiatry Research, 28*, 193–213.

Camacho-Gomez, M., & Castellvi, P. (2020). Effectiveness of family intervention for preventing relapse in first-episode psychosis until 24 months of follow-up: a systematic review with meta-analysis of randomized controlled trials. *Schizophrenia Bulletin, 46*, 98–109.

Cechnicki, A., Bielanska, A., Hanuszkiewicz, I., & Daren, A. (2013). The predictive validity of Expressed Emotions (EE) in schizophrenia: A 20-year prospective study. *Journal of Psychiatric Research, 47*(2), 208–214. doi:10.1016/j.jpsychires.2012.10.004

Chen, F. P., & Greenberg, J. S. (2004). A positive aspect of caregiving: The influence of social support on caregiving gains for family members of relatives with schizophrenia. *Community Mental Health Journal, 40*(5), 423–435.

Cherry, M. G., Taylor, P. J., Brown, S. L., Rigby, J. W., & Sellwood, W. (2017). Guilt, shame and expressed emotion in carers of people with long-term mental health difficulties: A systematic review. *Psychiatry Research*. doi.org/10.1016/j.psychres.2016.12.056

Cherry, M. G., Taylor, P. J., Brown, S. L., Rigby, J. W., & Sellwood, W. (2018). Attachment, mentalization and expressed emotion in carers of people with long-term mental health difficulties. *BMC Psychiatry, 18*, 257. https://doi.org/10.1186/s12888-018-1842-4

Claxton, M., Onwumere, J., & Fornells-Ambrojo, M. (2017). Do family interventions improve outcomes in early psychosis? A systematic review and meta-analysis. *Frontiers in Psychology, 8, 371*. doi:10.3389/fpsyg.2017.00371

Docherty, N. M., St-Hilaire, A., Aakre, J. M., Segher, J. P., McCleery, A., & Divilb, M. (2011). Anxiety interacts with expressed emotion criticism in the prediction of psychotic symptom exacerbation. *Schizophrenia Bulletin, 37*(3), 611–618. doi:10.1093/schbul/sbp123

Dominguez-Marinez, T., Medina-Pradas, C., Kwapil, T. R., & Barrantes-Vidal, N. (2017). Relatives expressed emotion, distress and attributions in clinical high risk and recent onset psychosis. *Psychiatry Research, 247*, 323–329.

Falloon, I. R. H., Boyd, J. L., & McGill, C. W. (1984). *Family care of schizophrenia: A problem-solving approach to the treatment of mental illness*. New York: Guilford Press.

Finnegan, D. (2011). *The effects of negative communication in psychosis: proof of principal and treatment development*. DClin Psy. Kings College London, UK.
Finnegan, D., Onwumere, J., Green, C., Freeman, D., Garety, P., & Kuipers, E. (2014). Negative communication in psychosis: Understanding pathways to poorer patient outcomes. *Journal of Nervous and Mental Disease, 202*(11), 829–883.
Fleischhacker, W. W., Arango, C., Arteel, P., Barnes, T. R., Carpenter, W., Duckworth, K., Galderisi, S., Halpern, L., Knapp, M., Marder, S. R., Moller, M., Sartorius, N., & Woodruff, P. (2014). Schizophrenia – time to commit to policy change. *Schizophrenia Bulletin, 40*, S165–S194.
Fridgen, G. J., Aston, J., Gschwandtner, U., Pflueger, M., Zimmermann, R., Studerus, E., Stieglitz, R. D., Riecher-Rössler, A. (2013). Help-seeking and pathways to care in the early stages of psychosis. *Social Psychiatry and Psychiatric Epidemiology, 48*, 1033–1043.
Galletly, C., Castle, D., Dark, F., Humberstone, V., Jablensky, A., Killackey, E., Kulkarni, J., McGorry, P., Nielssen, O., & Tran, N. (2016). Royal Australian and New Zealand College of Psychiatrists clinical practice guidelines for the management of schizophrenia and related disorders. *Australian and New Zealand Journal of Psychiatry, 50*, 410–472.
Garety, P. A., Kuipers, E., Fowler, D., Freeman, D., & Bebbington, P. E. (2001). A cognitive model of the positive symptoms of psychosis. *Psychological Medicine, 31*, 189–195.
Gayer-Anderson, C., & Morgan, C. (2013). Social networks, support and early psychosis: A systematic review. *Epidemiology and Psychiatric Sciences, 22*(2), 131–146. doi:10.1017/S2045796012000406
Gonzalez-Blanch, C., Gleeson, J. F., Cotton, S. M., Crisp, K., McGorry, P. D., & Alvarez-Jimenez, M. (2015). Longitudinal relationship between expressed emotion and cannabis misuse in young people with first-episode psychosis. *European Psychiatry, 30*, 20–25.
Gross, J. J. (2001). Emotion regulation in adulthood: Timing is everything. *Current Directions in Psychological Science, 10*(6), 214–219. http://dx.doi.org/10.1111/1467-8721.00152
Gross, J. J. (2002). Emotion regulation: Affective cognitive and social consequences. *Psychophysiology, 39*(3), 281–291.
Gross, J. J., & John, O. P. (2003). Individual differences in two emotion regulation processes: Implications for affect, relationships and well-being. *Journal of Personality and Social Psychology, 85*(2), 348–362.
Gupta, S., Isherwood, G., Jones, K., & Van Impe, K. (2015). Assessing health status in informal schizophrenia caregivers compared with health status in non-caregivers and caregivers of other conditions. *BMC Psychiatry, 15*, 162.
Gurak, K., & Wesiman De Mamani, A. (2017). Caregiver expressed emotion and psychiatric symptoms in African-Americans with schizophrenia: An attempt to understand the paradoxical relationship. *Family Process, 56*, 476–486.
Hall, P., & Tarrier, N. (2003). The cognitive behavioural treatment of low self-esteem in psychotic patients: A pilot study. *Behavior Research and Therapy, 41*(3), 317–322.
Hamaie, Y., Ohmuro, N., Katsura, M., Obara, C., Kikuchi, T., Ito, F., Miyakoshi, T., Matsuoka, H., & Matsumoto, K. (2016). Criticism and depression among the caregivers of at-risk mental state and first-episode psychosis patients. *PLoS One, 11*, e0149875.
Hayes, L., Hawthorne, G., Farhall, J., O'Hanlon, B., & Harvey, C. (2015). Quality of life and social isolation among caregivers of adults with schizophrenia: Policy and outcomes. *Community Mental Health Journal, 51*(5), 591–597. doi:10.1007/s10597-015-9848
Hayes JF, Marston L, Walters K, King MB & Osborn, DPJ (2017). Mortality gap for people with bipolar disorder and schizophrenia: UK-based cohort study 2000–2014. *The British Journal of Psychiatry, 211*(3), 175–181. doi: 10.1192/bjp.bp.117.202606

Hesse, K., Kriston, L., Mehl, S., Wittorf, A., Wiedemann, W., Wolwer, W., & Klingberg, S. (2015). The vicious cycle of family atmosphere, interpersonal self-concepts and paranoia in schizophrenia: A longitudinal study. *Schizophrenia Bulletin*, *41*, 1403–1412.

Hooley, J. M., & Campbell, C. (2002). Control and controllability: Beliefs and behaviour in high and low expressed emotion relatives. *Psychological Medicine*, *32*(6), 1091–1099.

Hsiao, C-Y. & Tsai, Y-F. (2014). Caregiver burden and satisfaction in families of individuals with schizophrenia. *Nursing Research*, *63*, 260–269.

Ince, P., Haddock, G., & Tai, S. (2016). A systematic review of the implementation of recommended psychological interventions for schizophrenia: Rates, barriers, and improvement strategies. *Psychology and Psychotherapy: Theory Research and Practice*, *89*, 324–350.

Jansen, J. E., Gleeson, J., & Cotton, S. (2015). Towards a better understanding of caregiver distress in early psychosis: A systematic review of the psychological factors involved. *Clinical Psychology Review*, *35*, 56–66.

Jansen, J. E., Lysaker, P. H., Harder, S., Haahr, U. H., Lyse, H. G., Pedersen, M. B., . . . Simonsen, E. (2014). Positive and negative caregiver experiences in first-episode psychosis: Emotional overinvolvement, wellbeing and metacognition. *Psychology and Psychotherapy: Theory Research and Practice*, *87*(3), 298–310.

Jongsma, H. E., Turner, C., Kirkbride, J. B., & Jones, P. B. (2019). International incidence of psychotic disorders, 2002–17: A systematic review and meta-analysis. *The Lancet Public Heath*, *4*, e229–e244.

Kageyama, M., & Solomon, P. (2018). Characteristics of parents with high expressed emotion and related factors: A study of parents of adults with schizophrenia. *The Journal of Nervous and Mental Disease*, *206*(12), 955–961. doi:10.1097/NMD.0000000000000902

Kageyama, M., Solomon, P., Kita, S., Nagata, S., Yokoyama, K., Nakamura, Y., . . . Fujii, C. (2016). Factors related to physical violence experienced by parents of persons in Japan. *Psychiatry Research*, *243*, 439–445.

Kingston, C., Onwumere, J., Keen, N., Ruffell, T., & Kuipers, E. (2016). Post traumatic symptoms in caregivers of people with psychosis and associations with caregiving experiences. *Journal of Trauma & Dissociation*, *17*(3), 307–321. doi.org/10.1080/15299732.2015.1089969

Koutra, K., Triliva, S., Roumeliotaki, T., Basta, M., Simos, P., Lionis, C., & Vgontzas, A. N. (2015). Impaired family functioning in psychosis and its relevance to relapse: A two year follow up study. *Comprehensive Psychiatry*, *62*, 1–12. doi.org/10.1016/j.comppsych.2015.06.006

Kreyenbuhl, J., Buchanan, R. W., Dickerson, F. B., & Dixon, L. B. (2010). The schizophrenia Patient Outcomes Research Team (PORT): Updated treatment recommendations 2009. *Schizophrenia Bulletin*, *36*(1), 94–103.

Kuipers, E., Bebbington, P., Dunn, G., Fowler, D., Freeman, D., Watson, P., Hardy, A., Garety, P. (2006). Influence of carer expressed emotion and affect on relapse in non-affective psychoses. *British Journal of Psychiatry*, *188*, 173–179.

Kuipers, E., Leff, J., & Lam, D. (2002). *Family work for schizophrenia: A practical guide* (2nd ed.). London: Gaskell.

Kuipers, E., Onwumere, J., & Bebbington, P. (2010). A cognitive model of caregiving in psychosis. *The British Journal of Psychiatry*, *196*, 259–265. doi:10.1192/bjp.bp.109.070466

Kuipers, E., Watson, P., Onwumere, J., Bebbington, P., Dunn, G., Weinman, J., Fowler, D., Freeman, D., Hardy, A., & Garety, P. (2007). Discrepant illness perceptions affect expressed emotion in people with psychosis and their carers. *Social Psychiatry and Psychiatric Epidemiology*, *42*, 277–283.

Lee, G., Barrowclough, C., & Lobban, F. (2014). Positive affect in the family environment protects against relapse in first-episode psychosis. *Social Psychiatry Psychiatric Epidemiology, 49*(3), 367–376. doi:10.1007/s00127-013-0768-x

Legg L., Weir C.J., Langhorne P., Smith L.N., Stott D.J. (2013). Is informal caregiving independently associated with poor health? A population-based study. *Journal of Epidemiology and Community Health, 67*, 95–97.

López, S. R., Hipke, K. N., Polo, A. J., Jenkins, J. H., Karno, M., & Vaughn, C. (2004). Ethnicity, expressed emotion, attributions, and course of schizophrenia: Family warmth matters. *Journal of Abnormal Psychology, 113*, 428–439.

Lucksted A., Stevenson J., Nossel I., Drapalski A., Piscitelli S., Dixon L.B. (2018) Family member engagement with early psychosis specialty care. *Early Intervention in Psychiatry, 12*(5), 922–927. doi: 10.1111/eip.12403.

Magliano, L., Fiorillo, A., De Rosa, C., Malangone, C., Maj, M., & National Mental Health Working Group. (2005). Family burden in long-term diseases: A comparative study in schizophrenia vs. physical disorders. *Social Science and Medicine, 61*(2), 313–322.

Marom, S., Munitz, H., Jones, P. B., Weizman, A., & Hermesh, H. (2005). Expressed emotion: Relevance to rehospitalisation in schizophrenia over 7 years. *Schizophrenia Bulletin, 31*(3), 751–758.

McCann, T. V., Lubman, D. I., & Clark, E. (2011). First-time primary caregivers' experience of caring for young adults with first-episode psychosis. *Schizophrenia Bulletin, 37*(2), 381–388.

Mittendorfer-Rutz, E., Rahman, S., Tanskanen, A., Majak, M., Mehtälä, J., Hoti, F., Jedenius, E., Enkusson, D., Level, A., Sermon, J., Taipale, H., & Tiihonen, J. (2019). Burden of parents of patients with schizophrenia: A nationwide comparative study of parents of offspring with rheumatoid arthritis, multiple sclerosis, epilepsy, and healthy controls. *Schizophrenia Bulletin, 18*, 794–803.

National Institute for Health and Care Excellence. (2014). *Psychosis and schizophrenia in adults: Treatment and management.* Clinical Guideline 178. London: NICE.

Norman, R., Lecomte, T., Addington, D., & Anderson, E. (2017). CPA treatment guidelines on psychosocial treatment of schizophrenia in adults. *Canadian Journal of Psychiatry/La Revue Canadienne de Psychiatrie*, 1–7. doi:10.1177/0706743717719894

Norman, R. M. G., Malla, A. K., Manchanda, R., Harricharan, R., Takhar, J., & Northcott, S. (2005). Social support and three-year symptom and admission outcomes for first episode psychosis. *Schizophrenia Research, 80*, 227–234.

O'Brien, M. P., Gordon, J. L., Bearden, C. E., López, S. R., Kopelowicz, A., & Cannon, T. D. (2006). Positive family environment predicts improvement in symptoms and social functioning among adolescents at imminent risk for onset of psychosis. *Schizophrenia Research, 81*(2–3), 269–275. doi:10.1016/j.schres.2005.10.005

O'Brien, M. P., Zinberg, J. L., Bearden, C. E., López, S. R., Kopelowicz, A., Daley, M., & Cannon, T. D. (2008). Parent attitudes and parent adolescent interaction in families of youth at risk for psychosis and with recent-onset psychotic symptoms. *Early Intervention in Psychiatry, 2*, 268–276.

O'Driscoll, C., Sener, S. B., Angmark, A., & Shaikh, M. (2019). Caregiving processes and expressed emotion in psychosis, a cross-cultural, meta-analytic review. *Schizophrenia Research.* https://doi.org/10.1016/j.schres.2019.03.020

Onwumere, J., Grice, S., Garety, P., Bebbington, P.,Dunn, G,Freeman, D., Fowler, D & Kuipers, E (2014). Caregiver reports of patient-initiated violence in psychosis. *Canadian Journal of Psychiatry, 59*(7), 376–384.

Onwumere, J., Grice, S., & Kuipers, E. (2016). Delivering cognitive-behavioural family interventions for schizophrenia: "Service systems must aim at supporting recovery in the whole family" (Jansen 2014 p. 13). *Australian Psychologist*, (51), 52–61.

Onwumere, J., Kuipers, E., Bebbington, P., Dunn, G., Fowler, D., Freeman, D. E., Watson, P., & Garety, P. (2008). Care-giving and illness beliefs in the course of psychotic illness. *Canadian Journal of Psychiatry, 53*, 460–468.

Onwumere, J., Kuipers, E., Bebbington, P., Dunn, G., Freeman, D., Fowler, D., & Garety, P. (2009). Patient perceptions of caregiver criticism in psychosis: Links with patient and caregiver functioning. *Journal of Nervous and Mental Disease, 197*, 85–91.

Onwumere, J., Kuipers, E., Bebbington, P., Dunn, G., Freeman, D., Fowler, D., & Garety, P. (2011). Coping styles in carers of people with recent and long-term psychosis. *Journal of Nervous and Mental Disease, 199*, 423–424.

Onwumere, J., Lotey, G., Schulz, J., Afsharzadegan, R., Harvey, R., Chu Man, L., Kuipers, E., & Raune, D. (2017). Burnout in early course psychosis caregivers: the role of illness beliefs and coping styles. *Early Intervention in Psychiatry, 11*, 237–243.

Onwumere J. Zhou Z, Kuipers E (2018). Informal caregiving in psychosis: reviewing the impact of patient-initiated violence. *Frontiers in Psychology, 9*, 1530. https://doi.org/10.3389/fpsyg.2018.01530

Palumbo, C., Volpe, U., Matanov, A., Priebe, S., & Giacco, D. (2015). Social networks of patients with psychosis: A systematic review. *BMC Research Notes, 8*, 560. doi:10.1186/s13104-015-1528-7

Pelayo-Terán, J. M., Gajardo Galán, V. G., de la Ortiz-García de la Foz, V., Martínez-García, O., Tabarés-Seisdedos, R., Crespo-Facorro, B., & Ayesa-Arriola, R. (2017). Rates and predictors of relapse in first-episode non-affective psychosis: A 3-year longitudinal study in a specialized intervention program (PAFIP). *European Archives of Psychiatry and Clinical Neuroscience, 267*, 315–323.

Perlick, D.A., Hohenstein, J.M., Clarkin, J.F., Kaczynski, R. & Rosenheck, R.A. (2005). Use of mental health and primary care services by caregivers of patients with bipolar disorder: a preliminary study. *Bipolar Disorders, 7*, 126–135.

Pharoah, F., Mari, J., Rathbone, J., & Wong, W. (2010). Family intervention for schizophrenia. *Cochrane Database Systematic Review*, (12), CD000088. doi:10.1002/14651858.CD000088.pub2

Poon, A. W. C., Curtis, J., Ward, P., Lonergan, C., & Lappin, J. (2018). Physical and psychological health of carers of young people with first episode psychosis. *Australasian Psychiatry, 26*(2), 184–188.

Ran, M. S., Chui, C. H. K., Wong, I. Y-L., Mao, W. J., Lin, F. R., Liu, B., & Chan, C. L. (2016). Family caregivers and outcome of people with schizophrenia in rural China: 14-year follow-up study. *Social Psychiatry and Psychiatric Epidemiology, 16*, 513–520.

Revier, C. J., Reininghaus, U., Dutta, R., Fearon, P., Murray, R. M., Doody, G. A., Croudace, T., Dazzan, P., Heslin, M., Onyejiaka, A., Kravariti, E., Lappin, J., Lomas, B., Kirkbride, J. B., Donoghue, K., Morgan, C., & Jones, P. B. (2015). Ten-year outcomes of first-episode psychoses in the MRC AESOP-10 study. *Journal of Nervous and Mental Disease, 203*, 379–386.

Robinson, D., Woerner, M. G., Alvir, J. M., Bilder, R., Goldman, R., Geisler, S., Koreen, A., Sheitman, B., Chakos, M., Mayerhoff, D., & Lieberman, J. A. (1999). Predictors of relapse following response from a first episode of schizophrenia or schizoaffective disorder. *Archives of General Psychiatry, 56*, 241–247.

Rosenfarb, I. S., Bellack, A. S., & Aziz, N. (2006). Family interactions and the course of schizophrenia in African American and White patients. *Journal of Abnormal Psychology, 115*, 112–120.

Roth, A. D., & Pilling, S. (2013). *A competence framework for psychological interventions for people with psychosis and bipolar disorder*. Retrieved June 19, 2018, from www.ucl.ac.uk/pals/research/clinical-educational-and-health-psychology/research-groups/core/competence-frameworks-10

Rylands, A. J., McKie, S., Elliot, R., Deakin, J. F. W., & Tarrier, N. (2011). A functional magnetic resonance imaging paradigm of expressed emotion in schizophrenia. *Journal of Nervous and Mental Disease, 199*, 25–29.

Sadath, A., Muralidhar, D., Varambally, S., Gangadhar, B. N., & Rose, J. R. (2017). Do stress and support matter for caring? The role of perceived stress and social support on expressed emotion of persons with first episode psychosis. *Asian Journal of Psychiatry, 25*, 163–168.

The Schizophrenia Commission. (2012). *The abandoned illness: A report from the schizophrenia commission*. London: Rethink Mental Illness.
Schlosser, D. A., Zinberg, J. L., Loewy, R. L., Casey-Cannon, S., O'Brien, M. P., Bearden, C. E., Vinogradov, S., & Cannon, T. D. (2010). Predicting the longitudinal effects of the family environment on prodromal symptoms and functioning in patients at-risk for psychosis. *Schizophrenia Research, 118*, 69–75.
Shiraishi, N., & Reilly, J. (2019). Positive and negative impacts of schizophrenia on family caregivers: A systematic review and qualitative meta-summary. *Social Psychiatry and Psychiatric Epidemiology, 54*, 277–290.
Smith, B., Fowler, D. G., Freeman, D., Bebbington, P., Bashforth, H., Garety, P., Dunn, G., & Kuipers, E. (2006). Emotion and psychosis: Links between depression, self-esteem, negative schematic beliefs and delusions and hallucinations. *Schizophrenia Research, 86*, 181–188.
Smith, L., Onwumere, J., Craig, T & Kuipers E (2018). Caregiver correlates of patient-initiated violence in early psychosis. *Psychiatry Research, 270*, 412–417.
Smith, L., Onwumere, J., Craig, T. & Kuipers E. (2019). A role for poor sleep in determining distress in caregivers of individuals with early psychosis. *Early Intervention in Psychiatry, 13*(3), 613–618 DOI: 10.1111/eip.12538
Smith, L., Onwumere, J., Craig, T., McManus, S., Bebbington, P., & Kuipers, E. (2014). Mental and physical illness in caregivers: Results from an English national survey sample. *The British Journal of Psychiatry, 205*(3), 197–203.
Sündermann, O., Onwumere, J., Kane, F., Morgan, C., & Kuipers, E. (2014). Social networks and support in first episode psychosis: Exploring the role of loneliness and anxiety. *Social Psychiatry and Psychiatric Epidemiology, 49*(3), 359–366. doi:10.1007/s00127-013-0754-3
Tomlinson, E., Onwumere, J., & Kuipers, E. (2014). Distress and negative experiences of the care-giving relationship in early psychosis-does social cognition play a role? *Early Intervention in Psychiatry, 8*(3), 253–260. doi:10.1111/eip.12040
Tompson, M. C., Goldstein, M. J., Lebell, M. B., Mintz, L. I., Marder, S. R., & Mintz, J. (1995). Schizophrenic-patients' perceptions of their relatives' attitudes. *Psychiatry Research, 57*(2), 155–167.
van Ments, M. (1999). *The effective use of role-play: Practical techniques for improving learning* (2nd ed.). London: Kogan Page Limited.
Vaughn, C. E., & Leff., J. P. (1976). The measurement of expressed emotion in families of psychiatric patients. *British Journal of Social and Clinical Psychology, 15*(2), 157–165.
Velthorst, E., Fett, A. J., Reichenberg, A., Perlman, G., van Os, J., Bromet, E. J., & Kotov, R. (2017). The 20-year longitudinal trajectories of social functioning in individuals with psychotic disorders. *American Journal of Psychiatry, 174*, 1075–1085.
Weintraub, M. J., Hall, D. L., Carbonella, J. Y., Weisman De Manani, A., & Hooley, J. (2017). Integrity of literature on expressed emotion and relapse in patients with schizophrenia verified by a p-Curve analysis. *Family Process, 56*(2), 436–444. doi:10.1111/famp.12208
Weintraub, M. J., Weisman de Mamani, A., Villano, W. J., Evans, T. C., Millman, Z. B., Hooley, J. M., & Timpano, K. R. (2019). Affective and physiological reactivity to emotional comments in individuals at elevated risk for psychosis. *Schizophrenia Research, 206*, 428–435.
Wood, H., Cupitt, C., & Lavender, T. (2015). The experience of cognitive impairment in people with psychosis. *Clinical Psychology and Psychotherapy, 22*(3), 193–207. doi:10.1002/cpp.1878
Zipursky, R. B., Menezes, N. M., & Streiner, D. L. (2014). Risk of symptom recurrence with medication discontinuation in first-episode psychosis: A systematic review. *Schizophrenia Research, 152*(2–3), 408–414. doi:10.1016/j.schres.2013.08.001

3

Beneath the Surface of Expressed Emotion (EE)

The Clinical Relevance of Possible Mechanisms Underlying EE in Eating Disorders

Mima Simic, Tom Jewell, and Ivan Eisler

Expressed Emotion and Eating Disorder Research – A Historical Perspective

Empirical studies of expressed emotion (EE) and eating disorders have accumulated rapidly over the past 40 years (see Duclos, Vibert, Mattar, & Godart (2012) and Rienecke (2018) for recent reviews). While the history of EE is covered in detail in Chapter 1 (Rienecke & Le Grange), we consider it important to briefly revisit how the concept of EE first entered the eating disorder field. By matter of happenstance, the developers of EE, such as George Brown, Michael Rutter, Julian Leff, and Christine Vaughn, were working at the same time and place as some of the early researchers of family therapy for eating disorders (Gerald Russell, George Szmukler, Christopher Dare, and Ivan Eisler): the Institute of Psychiatry and Maudsley Hospital in London. These two research groups shared common interests in the fine-grained analysis of family interactions and the potential impact of such interactions on the course of recovery from mental illness. The early EE studies in schizophrenia are notable for the extent to which the researchers focused on observations of interactional patterns *between* family members. For example, in Brown, Monck, Carstairs, and Wing's (1962) seminal study of men with schizophrenia, the rating scales of the family interviews included not only the caregiver's behavior towards the patient but also the patient's behavior towards the caregiver. In other words, from the early days, EE was conceptualized as an interactional construct rather than just a measure of parental attitude or behavior. A further important aspect of the EE measure is that it combines precise operational definitions, with a significant degree of subtle judgment required to be made by raters of specific behaviors (e.g. the tone, speed and pitch of speech), which gives the measure a high degree of clinical salience. This, together with the interactional nature of the EE concept, made it of particular interest to the Maudsley eating disorders research group and their desire to integrate empirical rigor with meaningful clinical judgment (Eisler, Szmukler, & Dare, 1985; Eisler, Dare, & Szmukler, 1988; Dare, Eisler, Colahan, Crowther, & Asen, 1995).

Developments in the Measurement of EE

Despite the interactional nature of the early EE studies, the measurement of EE was eventually operationalized as a set of rating scales applied to the Camberwell Family Interview (CFI – Rutter & Brown, 1966), a somewhat misleadingly titled instrument given the fact that it was administered to key relatives *individually* rather than in a conjoint format to families. In the early studies, a key relative would be interviewed for five to six hours about the development of the patient's illness and the emotional climate between the relative and patient, such as the frequency of quarrels (Brown, Birley, & Wing, 1972). Later shortened to around one hour by Vaughn and Leff (1976), the CFI became the gold-standard instrument for the assessment of EE, yielding five dimensions: Critical Comments (CC), Hostility (H), Emotional Overinvolvement (EOI), Warmth (W), and Positive Remarks (PR). The CFI rating scales have also been used to rate both clinical and research conjoint family interviews (Berkowitz, 1987; Szmukler, Berkowitz, Eisler, Leff, & Dare, 1987; Hodes, Dare, Dodge, & Eisler, 1999). While generating rich information, the CFI was time-consuming to administer and code, which provided the impetus for the development of shorter measures. Of particular note, the Five-Minute Speech Sample (FMSS – Magaña, Goldstein, Karno, &

Miklowitz, 1986), in which a relative is asked to speak about their relative without interruption from the interviewer for five minutes, yields two dimensions: CC and EOI. The relative is coded as high in EE if at least one of the CC or EOI dimensions is high. Finally, various self-report measures have been developed, including the Level of Expressed Emotions (LEE – Cole & Kazarian, 1988), a patient-reported measure, and the parent-reported Family Questionnaire (FQ – Wiedemann, Rayki, Feinstein, & Hahlweg, 2002).

Despite the proliferation of shorter EE measures, there have been few reviews of these alternatives. Two reviews (Van Humbeeck, Van Audenhove, De Hert, Pieters, & Storms, 2002; Hooley & Parker, 2006) concluded that the development of alternatives to the CFI had been relatively unsuccessful, pointing for instance to the modest predictive power of the FMSS and self-report questionnaires and low interrater reliability for some of the observational scales. The alternative measures have generally focused only on two of the dimensions of the original EE scales, CC and EOI (and in some cases, only CC). Of the two, the EOI scale has been particularly difficult to translate to the shorter versions. Particular doubts have been raised about the applicability of the EOI construct when applied to children and adolescents. As Peris and Miklowitz (2015) have pointed out, what may be constraining behavior in a parent of an adult with schizophrenia may be developmentally appropriate in a parent of a child or adolescent with a mental health problem.

Given that the construct of EE was developed more than 50 years ago, in a particular geographical context, and with a particular patient group – men with schizophrenia in urban England – it is striking how widely applicable the measure has been across different diagnostic groups, diverse cultural contexts and different stages of the family life-cycle. At the same time, the breadth of application of the measure raises important questions about the construct validity of EE when applied unquestioningly in these diverse contexts. For instance, Bhugra and McKenzie (2003), in their overview of EE studies in different cultural contexts, highlight that while EE has been found to be applicable as a measure across a wide range of cultures, there is considerable variation in the rates of, for example, critical or emotionally involved behaviors, as well as their impacts, depending on the varied cultural expectations. Likewise, there are also gender differences in the manifestation of EE. When individuals develop a mental health problem, it is typically their mothers who spend more time with their child, and consequently, they are more exposed to their difficulties. It has also been recognized that women tend to be more expressive than men (Wager & Ochsner, 2005). Parental roles may also differ during treatment, with mothers usually taking a more active role in providing care. Social expectations of gendered parental roles may also influence how behaviors are experienced. For instance, in adolescents with anorexia nervosa (AN), Szmukler, Eisler, Russell, and Dare (1985) showed that while fathers generally made fewer Critical Comments than mothers, both paternal and maternal EE predicted engagement in treatment but at different levels of criticism.

The Interactional Nature of EE

Unlike most other measures of family functioning, EE is neither a self-rating of perceived family functioning nor a direct observational measure of family interaction but is a rating of a relative's response to questions about day-to-day family life in the context of living with a mental illness. The CFI explores the relative's experiences of living with and caring for someone with mental health problems and the impact this has on the family. The rating of the CFI is based, in part, on the reported interactions between the patient and the relative, but a key focus is also on the emotional, primarily non-verbal, aspects of the response during the interview. The interview assumes that the nature of negative affective exchanges between family members is bi-directional in the sense that they are both a response to the illness and may also be reinforcing or maintaining it.

As the emphasis in the concept of EE is interactive, its impact on the occurrence of illness, its course and treatment response need to be explored as belonging to the interaction that happens in the relational context between parents and their child. In other words, to understand the significance of EE in treatment, it is best viewed as a marker of an interactional process, or as Vaughn (1989) describes it, a measure of the "emotional temperature" of the family that has the potential to act as a stressor for both child and parent. The high-EE environment has the potential to trigger the child's biological responses (threat sensitivity, stress reactivity, and arousal), coupled with the child's psychological features (attachment patterns, cognitive appraisal) and temperament. By the same token, the parental emotional response to the emerging eating disorder in their child can be seen as a reflection of their own biological and temperamental predispositions and vulnerabilities, their own attachment patterns, and the related perceptions of their parental self-efficacy and the way these are challenged by the specific symptom presentations.

As Peris and Miklowitz (2015) point out, the stress that all children at times experience in the home environment may in many instances serve a positive function of helping them to learn to regulate emotions, develop an ability to mentalize, and manage their future behavioral responses effectively. The long-term impact of stressful experiences depends on a number of factors, including the child's genetically influenced predispositions, the frequency of anxiety-provoking events, and, importantly, how supportive the family environment is (Repetti, Taylor, & Seeman, 2002). In a chronically distressed family environment, stressful events are more likely to have a negative effect, leading children to become hypervigilant to potential threats and their ability to mentalize is compromised (Allen, Fonagy, & Bateman, 2008). This can be more pronounced in young people who, due to their previous experiences or temperament, are more sensitive and have a lower threshold to perceive situations or reactions from other people as potentially threatening, especially when the dominant emotion is anger or hostility.

The fear that is associated with an emerging psychiatric disorder that threatens the sense of safety and survival of self (both in the child and parents) activates the attachment system between the child and parent. Once the attachment pattern is evoked by the stress, the child will look for the availability of parents to respond with a matching, reciprocal, protective, and regulating response to his/her distress and emotional pain. If parents respond with hostility, criticism, or blame, this may create emotionally charged environments that exacerbate symptoms, which in turn may fuel negative parent–child interactions and interfere with healthy behavior management strategies. A high-EE response from parents has the potential to trigger reciprocal and escalating patterns of interactions, leading to the formation of a self-perpetuating vicious circle.

In summary, parental high EE in response to the developing mental illness may represent a maladaptive pattern of responding to a child's illness that simultaneously arouses the child's physiological and psychological reactions, especially if it occurs in a vulnerable child and in the absence of buffering factors like parental support (for an in-depth discussion, see Miklowitz, 2004).

A key question in understanding the role of EE in families in which someone is developing a mental health problem is why the pattern described earlier applies only in some families. While there are limited data on EE that pre-date the development of mental health problems, there are likely to be a combination of factors (1) that are specific to the child (symptom presentation, temperament, expressions of emotional vulnerability) (Simic et al., 2016); (2) that are predispositions in the parent (flexibility, locus of control, levels of anxiety or depression), which it has been suggested create a continuum of vulnerability to respond in a high-EE manner (Hooley & Gotlib, 2000); and (3) that characterize the nature of the pre-illness family relationships and attachment patterns.

Expressed Emotion and Eating Disorders

In the field of eating disorders, EE has been studied fairly extensively, including as a predictor of treatment engagement (Szmukler et al., 1985) or treatment outcome (e.g. van Furth et al., 1996), as a potential moderator of treatment outcome (see Jewell, Blessitt, Stewart, Simic, & Eisler, 2016a for discussion) and as a treatment target in caregiver studies (Hibbs, Rhind, Leppanen, & Treasure, 2015). The research includes studies that have investigated EE and changes in EE over the course of treatment in families receiving family therapy for adolescent AN (e.g. Allan, Le Grange, Sawyer, McLean, & Hughes, 2018; Eisler et al., 2000; Le Grange, Eisler, Dare, & Hodes, 1992; Le Grange, Hoste, Lock, & Bryson, 2011; Rienecke, Accurso, Lock, & Le Grange, 2016) as well as studies of adult patients and their carers (Goddard et al., 2011; Sepulveda et al., 2010).

Differences in EE Between Diagnostic Subgroups and Healthy Controls

It is worth noting that the overall levels of EE in eating disorders are generally low compared with schizophrenia (Szmukler et al., 1985; Le Grange, Eisler, Dare, & Hodes, 1992; Le Grange, Hoste, Lock, & Bryson, 2011). While this appears to be the case across the board, there is some evidence that there may be some differences according to diagnosis, with caregivers of patients with bulimia nervosa (BN) having been found in some studies to have somewhat higher rates of EE than patients with AN (Szmukler et al., 1985; Hoste & Le Grange, 2008; Rienecke, Sim, Lock, & Le Grange, 2016), although other studies have not found a difference (van Furth et al., 1996; Di Paola, Faravelli, & Ricca, 2010; Santonastaso, Saccon, & Favaro, 1997). In comparison with healthy control groups, most studies report no differences in levels of criticism (Blair, Freeman, & Cull, 1995), but some studies have found raised levels on the EOI scale (Blair et al., 1995; Kyriacou, Treasure, & Schmidt, 2008; Di Paola et al., 2010).

EE and the Severity and Stages of Eating Disorder

Research studies have shown that families scoring high on EE are more likely in families of patients with a longer duration of illness (Hoste, Labuschagne, Lock, & Le Grange, 2012; Szmukler et al., 1985) and more numerous eating disorder symptoms (Hedlund, Fichter, Quadflieg, & Brandl, 2003). Furthermore, a larger number of previous episodes of treatment was linked to a higher level of parental criticism in a mixed eating disorders sample (Santonastaso et al., 1997). These findings suggest that in the older subjects, with more severe illness of a longer duration coupled with a history of more frequent past treatments, the parental exhaustion and distress might have led to higher levels of criticism and rejection.

EE as a Predictor of Treatment Engagement and Compliance With Treatment

A range of studies have found EE to be a good predictor of compliance in regard to the type of treatment offered. Early studies of the Maudsley family therapy found that a high level of EE (particularly maternal criticism) toward the adolescent was highly predictive of poor engagement in family therapy, while patients who dropped out of individual therapy were more likely to have critical fathers (Szmukler et al., 1985). Other AN studies have confirmed the finding that raised levels of maternal criticism were associated with poor engagement in family therapy (Dare, Eisler, Russell, & Szmukler, 1990; Rienecke, Accurso, Lock, & Le Grange,

2016). Similarly, in a BN study of family therapy and guided self-help cognitive-behavioral therapy (Schmidt et al., 2007), patient-perceived maternal EE was higher in patients who did not want to involve their parents in the treatment (Perkins et al., 2005).

EE as a Predictor of Treatment Response and Outcome

There is a considerable literature highlighting the role of raised parental EE on the course and outcome of treatment in eating disorders with poorer results in AN studies both at the end of treatment and five year follow-up (Le Grange et al., 1992; Eisler et al., 2000; Eisler, Simic, Russell, & Dare, 2007) or smaller improvement in psychological functioning (Moulds et al., 2000). Similar findings were found in a BN population (Hedlund et al., 2003) and in a population of mixed disorders in which van Furth et al. (1996), who studied the role of EE in the course of illness in a mixed sample of adolescent eating disorders, concluded that maternal Critical Comments accounted for 28–34% of the variance in treatment outcome. More recently, Rienecke, Accurso, et al. (2016) found that patients with mothers rated high in hostility gained more weight in individual therapy than in family-based treatment. Interestingly, Le Grange et al. (2011), in a study of an adolescent AN population, found that parental warmth was associated with a better weight outcome.

EE as a Potential Moderator of Treatment Outcome

Perhaps the most pressing issue for theory and research is the need to explain findings suggesting that conjoint family treatment, in which family members are seen together in sessions, may either result in poorer treatment outcomes in families with high EE (Le Grange et al., 1992; Eisler et al., 2000; Eisler et al., 2007) or might even increase levels of EE (Le Grange et al., 1992; Allan et al., 2018). A trial by Eisler et al. (2000) comparing conjoint and separated formats of family therapy for adolescent AN found no differences in outcome except for high-EE families, which fared better in separated sessions. This difference in outcome was still evident at five-year follow-ups (Eisler et al., 2007). Although in this study there were no overall differences in primary outcomes between separate and conjoint family therapy, there were some important differences in secondary outcomes. At a family level, the adolescents in the conjoint treatment arm rated their families as having become more flexible, while those in the separated treatment perceived the opposite, that is, that their families had become more rigid. Somewhat surprisingly, the conjoint treatment also proved to be more effective in bringing about change on a range of individual psychological measures including mood, obsessionality, and ED cognitions (Eisler et al., 2000; Dare, Chania, Eisler, Hodes, & Dodge, 2000).

More recently, Le Grange et al. (2016) conducted a similar study in adolescent AN, comparing conjoint family therapy, using the family-based treatment (FBT) manual (Lock & Le Grange, 2013), with parent-focused therapy (PFT). In the latter treatment, adolescents spent up to ten minutes talking with a nurse who weighed them, prior to the adolescent's parents then meeting for 50 minutes with a therapist who delivered treatment with a similar focus to FBT. In this study, adolescents who received PFT achieved better treatment outcomes at end-of-treatment than families receiving conjoint FBT, although the difference between treatments was not statistically significant at 6- or 12-month follow up. In a later secondary analysis of data from this study, Allan et al. (2018) found different patterns of change in EE between the two treatments. PFT was associated with a decrease in maternal criticism regardless of treatment outcome, whereas FBT was associated with increases in maternal criticism. The study authors also report that adolescents of mothers who demonstrated an increase in EE, or remained high in EE, were less likely to remit compared with adolescents for whom EE decreased or remained low.

EE as a Potential Target of Treatment

In addition to the family therapy studies with children and adolescents already described, a number of studies have investigated treatments aimed at carers of mainly adult patients. These included a range of interventions (skills and psychoeducational workshops, face-to face or online guided self-help) which were aimed at reducing carer distress and burden and influencing a range of carer behaviors, including reducing EE. A systematic review and meta-analysis indicate that such interventions can be effective and reduce carer burden and distress and lower EE (Hibbs et al., 2015), although the impact of such changes on patient outcomes is at present less clear.

An important caveat in attempting to interpret the above findings is that within the eating disorder field, there is substantial heterogeneity in how EE has been measured and reported (Duclos et al., 2012; Jewell et al., 2016a). For instance, while some studies have collapsed their data from several EE dimensions into a single categorical variable (e.g. Rienecke, Accurso, et al., 2016), others have used each separately as a continuous variable (e.g. van Furth et al., 1996), and several studies use only the Criticism dimension to inform their high- or low-EE classification (e.g. Eisler et al., 2000; Le Grange et al., 1992; Hodes et al., 1999). The classification of high and low EE has used a wide range of cut-off points for the number of criticisms rated in individual or family interviews, from >6 (e.g. Szmukler et al., 1985) as used in studies of schizophrenia down to >1 (e.g. Le Grange et al., 1992, 2011). In applying the FMSS ratings, some studies have included borderline ratings of criticism (i.e. dissatisfaction rather than outright criticism) (Rein et al., 2006), while others have not (Uehara, Kawashima, Goto, Tasaki, & Someya, 2001). Similarly, in the ratings of EOI, some have excluded "positive" aspects of parental involvement (high levels of praise, high levels of details about child's history or statements of loving attitudes) (van Furth, van Strien, van Son, & Van Engeland, 1993), while others have included them (Duclos et al., 2018; Allan et al., 2018; Rein et al., 2006) as defined by the scale developers.

Caution is also needed in adopting the conceptualization from the study of adults suffering from schizophrenia to other clinical populations. As mentioned earlier, this applies in particular to the concept of EOI (Peris & Miklowitz, 2015), which needs to be recalibrated when applied to a potentially life-threatening illness such as AN and understood in relation to multiple contexts, including eating disorder diagnosis and severity, culture, and gender. At the very least, the criteria by which EOI is rated would need to be adjusted to consider the developmental needs of the young person. Caution is also needed in adopting the categorical research definitions of high or low EE as "diagnostic" markers in clinical practice. The choice of very low cut-points for categorizing families as high or low on criticism may be justified at a group level in a research context, but it should not be automatically assumed that a single critical comment in a clinical family interview should define the family as high EE.

This heterogeneity, along with a lack of consistent reporting of findings for each EE dimension, may have obscured important relationships between specific dimensions and eating disorder outcomes and complicated the ease with which research findings can be understood. Before considering the clinical implications of the research findings, we put forward a theoretical framework of our understanding of how the temperamental, neurobiologically driven predisposing traits interact in some families with the emerging eating disorder leading to the specific dynamic of high-EE families.

Towards a Neurobiologically Informed Theory of Expressed Emotion and Eating Disorders

Frequent experiences of sustained and uncontrollable stress in the absence of protective influences provide one framework for understanding how a high-EE family environment interacts with individual biological vulnerabilities to increase the risk of illness, its reoccurrence and/or maintenance. In addition, the child's response to familial EE may also inform an understanding of how EE affects the course of eating disorders.

We propose that the concept of EE must be integrated both with systemic theory and the emerging evidence on the neurobiology of eating disorders (Frank et al., 2019; Eisler, 2005). Two principles are fundamental to our conceptualization. First, EE is an *interactional* phenomenon, in which patient behaviors and symptomatology and carer behaviors are mutually influencing of each other (Treasure & Schmidt, 2013). Second, a *shared genetic pool* within families results in common traits and common vulnerabilities, such as sensitivity to rejection, which can exacerbate distress and negative interactional cycles (Watson et al., 2019).

In Figure 3.1, we set out these ideas in diagrammatic form. At the start of treatment, the interactional, bidirectional relationship between eating disorder symptoms and carer EE is already present. Their impact on treatment will in part be mediated by temperamental traits that may be influenced by shared familial traits. Higher levels of threat sensitivity that includes *rejection sensitivity* (Cardi, Matteo, Corfield, & Treasure,

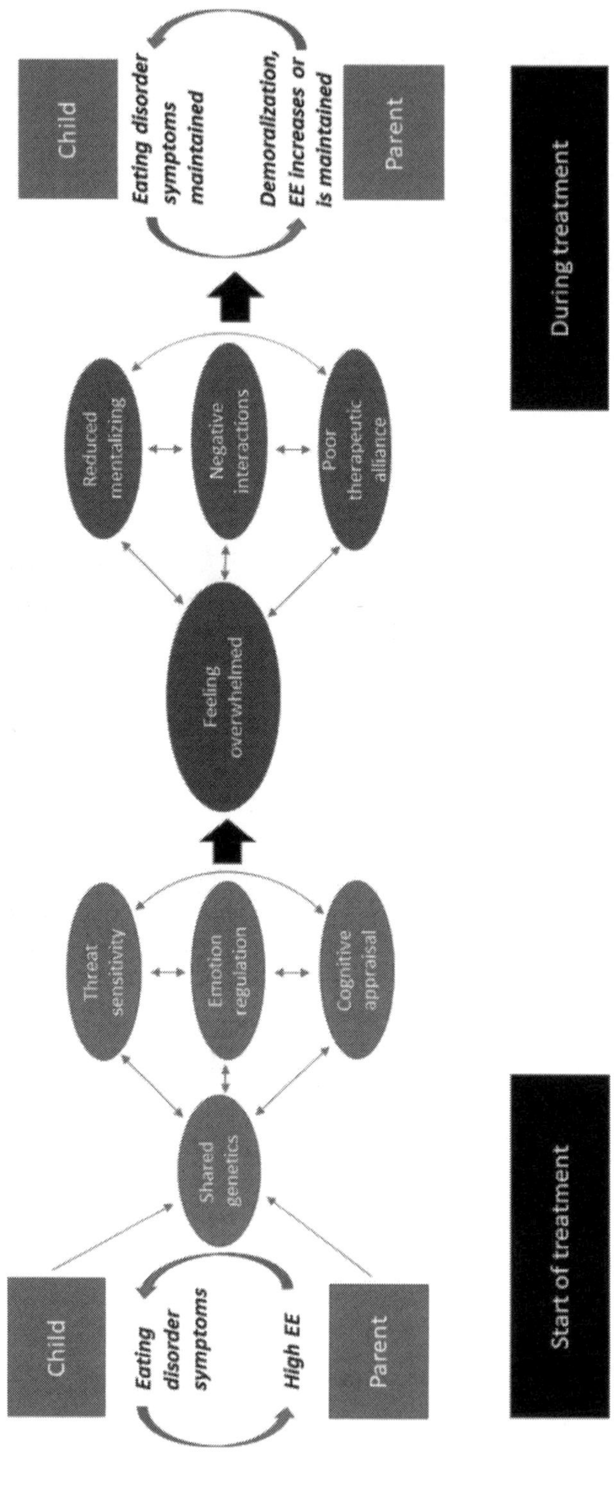

Figure 3.1 Theoretical model for role of high expressed emotion in the eating disorder treatment process

2013), attentional bias towards negative faces, associated with lower sensitivity to reward, is one mechanism by which EE may result in greater distress for both patients and carers.

Affect regulation processes are central to the interplay between EE and eating disorder symptoms. There is now substantial evidence of affect regulation difficulties within eating disorders, such as increased emotion suppression and avoidance in AN (Oldershaw, Lavender, Sallis, Stahl, & Schmidt, 2015; Oldershaw, Startup, & Lavender, 2019). Less well explored are the links between carer EE and affect regulation. We propose that *affect regulation processes* underlie both patient and carer responses: eating disorder-related behaviors exhibited by the patient can generate strong emotional responses in the carer such as anxiety, feelings of self-blame, or worthlessness (Besharat, Eisler, & Dare, 2001; Whitney & Eisler, 2005), which may lead to attempts to regulate such emotions through behaviors such as criticism, blame or over-excessive control. This in turn elicits strong emotions in the child, whose eating disorder symptoms may have a function in regulating her/his emotions, such as avoidance of negative emotional states (Brockmeyer et al., 2012; Henderson, Fox, Trayner, & Wittkowski, 2019). EE behaviors on the part of carers may unintentionally contribute to the development of emotionally charged environments that exacerbate symptoms, which in turn may fuel negative parent–child interaction and become part of a self-perpetuating vicious circle.

Further mediating the interplay between symptoms and EE might be the processes of *mentalizing*, a broad construct that includes the ability to self-reflect and understand mental states of others and the interaction between these two (Fonagy, Gergely, Jurist, & Target, 2002). Evidence for difficulties with mentalizing in eating disorder samples abounds (e.g. Caglar-Nazali et al., 2014) across a wide range of dimensions, including theory of mind (Bora & Köse, 2016) and emotion recognition (Jewell et al., 2016b). Importantly, while such difficulties may potentially represent traits that predate the onset of illness (Oldershaw et al., 2019), such difficulties increase with starvation (Bora & Köse, 2016), meaning that the potential for misappraisal of intentions is increased for many people with an eating disorder. In addition, mentalization abilities are diminished or switched off by high arousal and feeling overwhelmed (Allen et al., 2008).

These processes have tangible effects on the course of treatment. First, an intense *state of distress and feeling overwhelmed* is likely to arise for patients and carers experiencing the vicious circle of high EE and eating disorder symptoms. *Negative interactions* are likely to develop, such as increased conflict between patient and carer, but crucially, these are not confined to the home environment and also play out in the treatment context. When treatment is delivered conjointly with patient and carer(s) and high EE is present, clinicians are also liable to experience affective arousal and mentalize less well. The risk is that in such circumstances, sessions can be characterized by patterns of criticism (some of which may be aimed at the clinician), blame and anger, with patients and carers leaving such sessions feeling uncontained by the therapist and lacking hope for recovery. There is evidence that high levels of EE at the start of treatment may be of particular importance by contributing to a *poor therapeutic alliance* (Rienecke, Richmond, & Lebow, 2016), and, as previously mentioned, high levels of EE at baseline may have an impact on long term outcome at five years, even in families in which the levels of EE had reduced by the end of one year of treatment (Eisler et al., 2007). The likely explanation of this finding is that high levels of negative affect in the early stages of treatment may have had a negative impact on the development of the therapeutic alliance, which is associated with treatment outcomes (Graves et al., 2017). Lack of progress in treatment can then lead to carer feelings of inadequacy and demoralization, which in turn fuel further emotional dysregulation, leading to an increase or maintenance of EE behaviors such as criticism. This in turn further entrenches the eating disorder symptoms.

In exploring the role of EE in the treatment of eating disorders, it is therefore important to consider not just the family but also the therapeutic system. The role of the therapist is crucial in managing the potential escalations of negative affect and the disruptive effect this may have on the effective engagement of the family in a working therapeutic alliance. For this to happen, the therapist needs to be self-reflective and able to continue to mentalize during the unremitting high distressed state of the family system, aiming to create a sense of safety and containment, validate difficult feelings and offer understanding for the mental states of each of the family members. If the family members perceive that they had been understood and their emotions are validated by the therapist, they may be more likely to feel a sense of containment. This may then enhance the therapeutic relationship, for instance, by helping to establish a shared sense of purpose (Friedlander, Escudero, Heatherington, & Diamond, 2011).

Low EE in Families

The main focus of this chapter has been the exploration of the evolution of the high-EE family dynamic in the context of eating disorders. We have paid relatively little attention to low EE in families, not least because there is little empirical data on what characterize low-EE families other than an absence of high EE features. Our understanding of how low-EE families are impacted by an eating disorder is much more limited, although it is likely that low-EE families are a heterogeneous group whose response to the developing eating disorder will be varied. This heterogeneity may be only partly captured by other EE dimensions such as Warmth or Positive Remarks (Le Grange et al., 2011).

Given the impact on families of caring for someone with an eating disorder (Whitney & Eisler, 2005) and the known association between EE and the level of burden and distress experienced by carers (Kyriacou et al., 2008; Rhind et al., 2016), it is in many ways surprising that levels of EE in these families are generally low. In many instances, this may be an indication of the general relational and caring strength and resilience of the family and explains why family interventions, particularly early on in the course of the illness, are effective. We hypothesize that, while the family may feel disabled by the eating disorder, if the underlying family relationships are essentially sound, effective engagement in treatment enables the reactivation of parenting and relational patterns that pre-date the illness and, together with the containment and support provided by the clinical team, allows the early behavioral change to happen. This behavioral change will be the key building block to begin the process of recovery.

However, while low-EE families in general engage more readily in family treatments than high-EE families, our clinical experience suggests this is not universally the case. In some low-EE parents, their biological or psychological predispositions, probably best described as alexithymia or overcontrol, mean that although they might feel inwardly extremely anxious or desperate, they are less likely to express outwardly negative emotions and make negative remarks. In addition, their expression of warmth might be diminished. The absence of criticism or blame may also be connected to the parent's appraisal of the eating disorder as an illness over which the young person does not have control. While this may avoid the pernicious spiral described earlier, in some parents, the appraisal of the eating disorder as uncontrollable may reinforce their sense of pessimism about recovery and negatively impact their perceptions of self-efficacy (Fox, Dean, & Whittlesea, 2017). The resulting sense of helplessness and despair, alongside feelings of guilt and self-blame, will be reinforced in some families by poor experiences of previous treatments, repeated hospitalizations or other factors such as additional mental health problems in the family or other adverse life events.

In this group of families, some of the interventions that are helpful with other families such as trying to instill hope, expressions of therapeutic optimism or emphasizing the positive role that families can play in the process of recovery can be counterproductive, as they may be experienced by the family as invalidating their experiences and feeling that the therapist does not understand the enormity of what they are facing.

The Clinical Implications of Research Findings on EE and Eating Disorders

We now have more than 30 years of research findings on the relevance of EE to treatment process and outcome in eating disorders. These findings have important implications for how we deliver eating disorders–focused family therapy and modifications or choices of treatment to better meet the needs of individual families. The EE findings suggest that treatment process issues have a significant impact on outcome and raise some crucial questions for the field. Why does conjoint treatment appear to increase parental EE in some families? How does the therapeutic process interact with higher parental EE, leading to poorer treatment engagement and poorer outcomes in adolescent eating disorders? When do we need to modify or change treatment if EE is high or increasing during treatment? What interventions can be used to reduce high-EE interactions? When is low EE an indication that the family feels so completely overwhelmed that a focus on parent-led behavioral change in the young person may stall and reinforce the parent's sense of failure? Do we sometimes persist too long with "more of the same", and what should we add or modify to overcome the impasse in these situations?

There are several ways of addressing such questions. The first might be to ensure that therapists have a repertoire of therapeutic techniques that aim to reduce high EE behaviors. This may include psychoeducation about eating disorders or externalization of the illness, which are assumed to reduce feelings of guilt and blame to make negative or hostile interactions less likely to occur (Eisler et al., 2016; Lock & Le Grange, 2013; Le Grange & Lock, 2009) or more targeted interventions such as circular questions exploring perceptions of links between anxiety and criticism (Eisler et al., 2016). More broadly, the EE findings could be used to identify contra-indications to relying on a conjoint family therapy approach and instead offering a separated or parent-focused therapy. Both strategies have their place but also have limitations.

In the separated forms of family therapy investigated in the Eisler et al. (2000) and Le Grange et al. (2016) studies, reducing parental EE was not a specific treatment focus. Nevertheless, in the Le Grange et al. (2016) study, adolescents receiving separated parent-focused treatment (PFT) did better at end-of-treatment, and their parents were more likely to reduce their EE than parents of adolescents who received conjoint therapy. This suggests that the treatment process in separated treatment had tangible differences from conjoint therapy, with different impacts on low-or high-EE interactions. This might point in the direction of avoiding a conjoint approach with high-EE families, but that, too, is not straightforward. The limitations of such an approach are (1) it assumes a robustness of the empirical findings to justify such choices, which is currently lacking, and (2) that findings are understood as applying to the treatment as a whole rather than to a specific aspect of the treatment process, again an assumption that is difficult to justify on current evidence. As described earlier, the Eisler et al. (2000) study also highlights that there may be advantages to the conjoint approach that may be lost if our decision tree for choice of treatment is determined purely by looking at overall treatment outcome.

More thought is also needed on how best to support the low-EE parents who feel too overwhelmed by the enormity of the task of having a central role in helping their children. Some families may benefit from more frequent sessions in the very early stage of treatment with a more instructive therapeutic stance that provides guidance for parents on how to manage problem situations at home. This may be necessary until parents build up trust in the therapy and confidence in their own resourcefulness. Additional support for parents in the context of a parent group (Nicholls & Yi, 2012), multi-family therapy (Eisler et al., 2016), or just a facilitated meeting with other parents (Rhodes et al., 2008) can help open new conversations with the family on how they can move forward.

We believe that the theoretical model we have presented in this chapter offers another option which is a more nuanced, contextualized approach to treatment modification. We have suggested earlier that conjoint treatment can sometimes lead to interactions within sessions that lead to high emotional arousal and attendant poorer mentalizing, particularly in families in which attachment representations are less secure (Jewell et al., 2016b). In some cases, this could lead to a situation in which the adolescent's apparent rejection of help leads to an increase in parental negativity and criticism, thereby fueling a vicious circle of the kind described earlier (see Figure 3.1). Importantly, separated treatment may offer parents in particular an opportunity to feel more supported and understood by the therapist, with sessions providing a more reflective space in which parents are more contained (Wallis et al., 2017).

If this formulation is correct, it suggests that clinicians and researchers should pay attention not only to the presence or absence of high EE but also to variables such as arousal, feelings of rejection, and mentalizing, which may influence the atmosphere of both treatment sessions and life at home. Crucially, therapists and supervisors need to reflect on the impact that an emotionally charged environment has on the therapist and how the therapist responds. This shifts the focus from simply trying to reduce high-EE behaviors of the parents to the mediating variables that we have proposed that may offer worthwhile treatment targets for a range of therapeutic interventions. Some of these may be delivered more effectively in separate sessions with parents and the young person, although once containment and improved mentalization have been achieved and sustained, conjoint sessions may be resumed to good effect. Therapeutic interventions focusing on identifying, understanding, and validating emotions would be highly congruent with addressing in treatment sensitivity to rejection, emotion regulation, and mentalization, which might in turn lead to better treatment outcomes. Reducing EE can and should be a direct treatment focus in some families, but the generally low rates of EE in eating disorder samples suggest that we need to expand our thinking about treatment targets towards constructs with broader salience. Further exploration of low EE is warranted to determine if the high levels of hopelessness and helplessness that are present might suppress the expression of warmth and reduce positive attachment interactions (Le Grange et al., 2011). When high EE is present, therapy should aim to help parents and young people develop skills to self-soothe and strategies to tolerate distress.

The importance of tolerating distress is particularly important in eating disorders given that exposure to fear is central to eating disorder treatment regardless of treatment modality (Murray et al., 2018) and that outside of the sessions, it will often be parents and carers who need to support patients. Treatment aims to expose patients to specific fears ranging from fear of gaining weight, eating adequate or regular amounts of food with increased content of carbohydrates and fats, limiting or stopping exercise, or having to eat regularly without bingeing or vomiting. If patients' habituation to fears is delayed or disrupted and they are continuously in a heightened state of stress, this will inadvertently and negatively impact the effectiveness of treatment interventions. Calm and compassionate responses and support from their parents is critical to allow them to have a safe space and sufficient time for the habituation to take place. This is a further mechanism by which EE may influence treatment outcome. However, we suggest that a limited focus on reducing parental EE is unlikely to succeed if it does not address the underlying factors that make high EE (or low expressed warmth) more likely – thus, an intervention that helps parents acquire skills to cope with anxiety and tolerate distress may be a crucial target by which EE can be reduced and parental ability to support their children to do the same increased.

Conclusion

In this chapter, we have outlined the need for a nuanced and critical understanding of the EE construct, suggesting that it requires some refinement for eating disorder populations, particularly adolescent ones.

We have proposed some theoretical ideas that may help to guide treatment and future research.

We believe that there are rich connections to be made between EE and broader research findings on eating disorders, neurobiology, temperament, and emotion regulation. To make progress, researchers first need to pay attention to the EE construct and its measurement, which may require the development of new measures or the adaptation of existing ones to collect more nuanced data and revisit the original aim of EE developers to incorporate the interactional context in the measure. Second, research is needed that builds on and refines theoretical models that can translate into treatment innovation (Pennesi & Wade, 2016). Future observational and experimental studies should measure EE at multiple time points during treatment, along with related constructs such as emotional regulation, to inform the modification of current treatments or the development of novel treatments. Interventions that target the lowering of EE and that investigate the mechanisms by which this can be achieved are particularly needed in the adolescent field. In the meantime, we strongly encourage clinicians to keep EE in mind in their efforts to modify and personalize treatment.

References

Allan, E., Le Grange, D., Sawyer, S. M., McLean, L. A., & Hughes, E. K. (2018). Parental expressed emotion during two forms of family-based treatment for adolescent anorexia nervosa. *European Eating Disorders Review*, *26*(1), 46–52.

Allen, J. G., Fonagy, P., & Bateman, A. W. (2008). *Mentalizing in clinical practice*. Washington, DC: American Psychiatric Pub.

Berkowitz, R. (1987). Rating expressed emotion from initial family therapy sessions (a pilot study). *Journal of Family Therapy*, *9*(1), 27–37.

Besharat, M. A., Eisler, I., & Dare, C. (2001). The Self-and Other-Blame Scale (SOBS): The background and presentation of a new instrument for measuring blame in families. *Journal of Family Therapy*, *23*(2), 208–223.

Bhugra, D., & McKenzie, K. (2003). Expressed emotion across cultures. *Advances in Psychiatric Treatment*, *9*(5), 342–348.

Blair, C., Freeman, C., & Cull, A. (1995). The families of anorexia nervosa and cystic fibrosis patients. *Psychological Medicine*, *25*(5), 985–993.

Bora, E., & Köse, S. (2016). Meta-analysis of theory of mind in anorexia nervosa and bulimia nervosa: A specific İmpairment of cognitive perspective taking in anorexia nervosa? *International Journal of Eating Disorders*, *49*(8), 739–740.

Brockmeyer, T., Holtforth, M. G., Bents, H., Kämmerer, A., Herzog, W., & Friederich, H. C. (2012). Starvation and emotion regulation in anorexia nervosa. *Comprehensive Psychiatry*, *53*(5), 496–501.

Brown, G. W., Birley, J. L., & Wing, J. K. (1972). Influence of family life on the course of schizophrenic disorders: A replication. *The British Journal of Psychiatry*, *121*(562), 241–258.

Brown, G. W., Monck, E. M., Carstairs, G. M., & Wing, J. K. (1962). Influence of family life on the course of schizophrenic illness. *British Journal of Preventive & Social Medicine, 16*, 55–68.

Caglar-Nazali, H. P., Corfield, F., Cardi, V., Ambwani, S., Leppanen, J., Olabintan, O., . . . Micali, N. (2014). A systematic review and meta-analysis of "systems for social processes" in eating disorders. *Neuroscience & Biobehavioral Reviews, 42*, 55–92.

Cardi, V., Matteo, R. D., Corfield, F., & Treasure, J. (2013). Social reward and rejection sensitivity in eating disorders: An investigation of attentional bias and early experiences. *The World Journal of Biological Psychiatry, 14*(8), 622–633.

Cole, J. D., & Kazarian, S. S. (1988). The level of expressed emotion scale: A new measure of expressed emotion. *Journal of Clinical Psychology, 44*(3), 392–397.

Dare, C., Chania, E., Eisler, I., Hodes, M., & Dodge, L. (2000). The Eating Disorder Inventory as an instrument to explore change in adolescents in family therapy for anorexia nervosa. *European Eating Disorders Review, 8*, 369–383.

Dare, C., Eisler, I., Colahan, C., Crowther, R., Sr., & Asen, E. (1995). The listening heart and the Chi-square: Clinical and empirical perceptions in the family therapy of anorexia nervosa. *Journal of Family Therapy, 17*, 19–45.

Dare, C., Eisler, I., Russell, G. F., & Szmukler, G. I. (1990). The clinical and theoretical impact of a controlled trial of family therapy in anorexia nervosa. *Journal of Marital and Family Therapy, 16*(1), 39–57.

Di Paola, F., Faravelli, C., & Ricca, V. (2010). Perceived expressed emotion in anorexia nervosa, bulimia nervosa, and binge-eating disorder. *Comprehensive Psychiatry, 51*(4), 401–405.

Duclos, J., Dorard, G., Cook-Darzens, S., Curt, F., Faucher, S., Berthoz, S., . . . Godart, N. (2018). Predictive factors for outcome in adolescents with anorexia nervosa: To what extent does parental expressed emotion play a role? *PloS One, 13*(7), e0196820.

Duclos, J., Vibert, S., Mattar, L., & Godart, N. (2012). Expressed emotion in families of patients with eating disorders: A review of the literature. *Current Psychiatry Reviews, 8*(3), 183–202.

Eisler, I. (2005). The empirical and theoretical base of family therapy and multiple family day therapy for adolescent anorexia nervosa. *Journal of Family Therapy, 27*(2), 104–131.

Eisler, I., Dare, C., Hodes, M., Russell, G., Dodge, E., & Le Grange, D. (2000). Family therapy for adolescent anorexia nervosa: The results of a controlled comparison of two family interventions. *The Journal of Child Psychology and Psychiatry and Allied Disciplines, 41*(6), 727–736.

Eisler, I., Dare, C., & Szmukler, G. I. (1988). What's happened to family interaction research? An historical account and a family systems viewpoint. *Journal of Marital and Family Therapy, 14*, 45–61.

Eisler, I., Simic, M., Hodsoll, J., Asen, E., Berelowitz, M., Connan, F., . . . Landau, S. (2016). A pragmatic randomised multi-centre trial of multifamily and single family therapy for adolescent anorexia nervosa. *BMC Psychiatry, 16*, 422.

Eisler, I., Simic, M., Russell, G. F., & Dare, C. (2007). A randomised controlled treatment trial of two forms of family therapy in adolescent anorexia nervosa: A five-year follow-up. *Journal of Child Psychology and Psychiatry, 48*(6), 552–560.

Eisler, I., Szmukler, G. I., & Dare, C. (1985). Systematic observation and clinical insight: Are they compatible? An experiment in recognizing family interactions. *Psychological Medicine, 15*, 173–188.

Fonagy, P., Gergely, G., Jurist, E. L., & Target, M. (2002). *Affect regulation, mentalization, and the development of the self.* New York: Other Press.

Fox, J. R., Dean, M., & Whittlesea, A. (2017). The experience of caring for or living with an individual with an eating disorder: A meta-synthesis of qualitative studies. *Clinical Psychology & Psychotherapy, 24*(1), 103–125.

Frank, G. K., DeGuzman, M. C., & Shott, M. E. (2019). Motivation to eat and not to eat: The psycho-biological conflict in anorexia nervosa. *Physiology & Behaviour, 206*, 185–190.

Friedlander, M. L., Escudero, V., Heatherington, L., & Diamond, G. M. (2011). Alliance in couple and family therapy. *Psychotherapy, 48*(1), 25.

Goddard, E., Macdonald, P., Sepulveda, A. R., Naumann, U., Landau, S., Schmidt, U., & Treasure, J. (2011). Cognitive interpersonal maintenance model of eating disorders: Intervention for carers. *The British Journal of Psychiatry, 199*(3), 225–231.

Graves, T. A., Tabri, N., Thompson-Brenner, H., Franko, D. L., Eddy, K. T., Bourion-Bedes, S., . . . Isserlin, L. (2017). A meta-analysis of the relation between therapeutic alliance and treatment outcome in eating disorders. *International Journal of Eating Disorders, 50*(4), 323–340.

Hedlund, S., Fichter, M. M., Quadflieg, N., & Brandl, C. (2003). Expressed emotion, family environment, and parental bonding in bulimia nervosa: A 6-year investigation. *Eating and Weight Disorders-Studies on Anorexia, Bulimia and Obesity, 8*(1), 26–35.

Henderson, Z. B., Fox, J. R., Trayner, P., & Wittkowski, A. (2019). Emotional development in eating disorders: A qualitative metasynthesis. *Clinical Psychology & Psychotherapy, 26*(4), 440–457.

Hibbs, R., Rhind, C., Leppanen, J., & Treasure, J. (2015). Interventions for caregivers of someone with an eating disorder: A meta-analysis. *International Journal of Eating Disorders, 48*(4), 349–361.

Hodes, M., Dare, C., Dodge, E., & Eisler, I. (1999). The assessment of expressed emotion in a standardised family interview. *Journal of Child Psychology and Psychiatry, 40*, 617–625.

Hooley, J. M., & Gotlib, I. H. (2000). A diathesis-stress conceptualization of expressed emotion and clinical outcome. *Applied and Preventive Psychology, 9*(3), 135–151.

Hooley, J. M., & Parker, H. A. (2006). Measuring expressed emotion: An evaluation of the shortcuts. *Journal of Family Psychology, 20*(3), 386.

Hoste, R. R., Labuschagne, Z., Lock, J., & Le Grange, D. (2012). Cultural variability in expressed emotion among families of adolescents with anorexia nervosa. *International Journal of Eating Disorders, 45*(1), 142–145.

Hoste, R. R., & Le Grange, D. (2008). Expressed emotion among white and ethnic minority families of adolescents with bulimia nervosa. *European Eating Disorders Review: The Professional Journal of the Eating Disorders Association, 16*(5), 395–400.

Jewell, T., Blessitt, E., Stewart, C., Simic, M., & Eisler, I. (2016a). Family therapy for child and adolescent eating disorders: A critical review. *Family Process, 55*(3), 577–594.

Jewell, T., Collyer, H., Gardner, T., Tchanturia, K., Simic, M., Fonagy, P., & Eisler, I. (2016b). Attachment and mentalization and their association with child and adolescent eating pathology: A systematic review. *International Journal of Eating Disorders, 49*, 354–373.

Kyriacou, O., Treasure, J., & Schmidt, U. (2008). Expressed emotion in eating disorders assessed via self-report: An examination of factors associated with expressed emotion in carers of people with anorexia nervosa in comparison to control families. *International Journal of Eating Disorders, 41*(1), 37–46.

Le Grange, D., Eisler, I., Dare, C., & Hodes, M. (1992). Family criticism and self-starvation: A study of expressed emotion. *Journal of Family Therapy, 14*(2), 177–192.

Le Grange, D., Hoste, R. R., Lock, J., & Bryson, S. W. (2011). Parental expressed emotion of adolescents with anorexia nervosa: Outcome in family-based treatment. *International Journal of Eating Disorders, 44*(8), 731–734.

Le Grange, D., Hughes, E. K., Court, A., Yeo, M., Crosby, R. D., & Sawyer, S. M. (2016). Randomized clinical trial of parent-focused treatment and family-based treatment for adolescent anorexia nervosa. *Journal of the American Academy of Child & Adolescent Psychiatry*, *55*(8), 683–692.

Le Grange, D., & Lock, J. (2009). *Treating bulimia in adolescents: A family-based approach*. New York: Guilford Press.

Lock, J., & Le Grange, D. (2013). *Treatment manual for anorexia nervosa: A family-based approach*. New York: Guilford Press.

Magaña, A. B., Goldstein, M. J., Karno, M., & Miklowitz, D. J. (1986). A brief method for assessing expressed emotion in relatives of psychiatric patients. *Psychiatry Research*, *17*(3), 203–212.

Miklowitz, D. J. (2004). The role of family systems in severe and recurrent psychiatric disorders: A developmental psychopathology view. *Development and Psychopathology*, *16*(3), 667–688.

Moulds, M. L., Touyz, S. W., Schotte, D., Beumont, P. J., Griffiths, R., Russell, J., & Charles, M. (2000). Perceived expressed emotion in the siblings and parents of hospitalized patients with anorexia nervosa. *International Journal of Eating Disorders*, *27*(3), 288–296.

Murray, S. B., Strober, M., Craske, M. G., Griffiths, S., Levinson, C. A., & Strigo, I. A. (2018). Fear as a translational mechanism in the psychopathology of anorexia nervosa. *Neuroscience & Biobehavioral Reviews*, *95*, 383–395.

Nicholls, D. E., & Yi, I. (2012). Early intervention in eating disorders: A parent group approach. *Early Intervention in Psychiatry*, *6*(4), 357–367.

Oldershaw, A., Lavender, T., Sallis, H., Stahl, D., & Schmidt, U. (2015). Emotion generation and regulation in anorexia nervosa: A systematic review and meta-analysis of self-report data. *Clinical Psychology Review*, *39*, 83–95.

Oldershaw, A., Startup, H., & Lavender, T. (2019). Anorexia nervosa and a lost emotional self: A psychological formulation of the development, maintenance, and treatment of anorexia nervosa. *Frontiers in Psychology*, *10*.

Pennesi, J. L., & Wade, T. D. (2016). A systematic review of the existing models of disordered eating: Do they inform the development of effective interventions? *Clinical Psychology Review*, *43*, 175–192.

Peris, T. S., & Miklowitz, D. J. (2015). Parental expressed emotion and youth psychopathology: New directions for an old construct. *Child Psychiatry & Human Development*, *46*(6), 863–873.

Perkins, S., Schmidt, U., Eisler, I., Treasure, J., Yi, I., Winn, S., . . . Berelowitz, M. (2005). Why do adolescents with bulimia nervosa choose not to involve their parents in treatment? *European Child and Adolescent Psychiatry*, *14*, 376–385.

Rein, Z., Perdereau, F., Curt, F., Jeammet, P., Fermanian, J., & Godart, N. (2006). Expressed emotion and anorexia nervosa: The validation of the five-minute speech sample in reference to the Camberwell family interview. *International Journal of Eating Disorders*, *39*(3), 217–223.

Repetti, R. L., Taylor, S. E., & Seeman, T. E. (2002). Risky families: Family social environments and the mental and physical health of offspring. *Psychological Bulletin*, *128*(2), 330.

Rhind, C., Salerno, L., Hibbs, R., Micali, N., Schmidt, U., Gowers, S., . . . Lo Coco, G. (2016). The objective and subjective caregiving burden and caregiving behaviours of parents of adolescents with anorexia nervosa. *European Eating Disorders Review*, *24*(4), 310–319.

Rhodes, P., Baillee, A., Brown, J., & Madden, S. (2008). Can parent-to-parent consultation improve the effectiveness of the Maudsley model of family-based treatment for anorexia nervosa? A randomized control trial. *Journal of Family Therapy*, *30*(1), 96–108.

Rienecke, R. D. (2018). Expressed emotion and eating disorders: An updated review. *Current Psychiatry Reviews*, *14*(2), 84–98.

Rienecke, R. D., Accurso, E. C., Lock, J., & Le Grange, D. (2016). Expressed emotion, family functioning, and treatment outcome for adolescents with anorexia nervosa. *European Eating Disorders Review*, *24*(1), 43–51.

Rienecke, R. D., Richmond, R., & Lebow, J. (2016). Therapeutic alliance, expressed emotion, and treatment outcome for anorexia nervosa in a family-based partial hospitalization program. *Eating Behaviors*, *22*, 124–128.

Rienecke, R. D., Sim, L., Lock, J., & Le Grange, D. (2016). Patterns of expressed emotion in adolescent eating disorders. *Journal of Child Psychology and Psychiatry*, *57*(12), 1407–1413.

Rutter, M., & Brown, G. W. (1966). The reliability and validity of measures of family life and relationships in families containing a psychiatric patient. *Social Psychiatry*, *1*(1), 38–53.

Santonastaso, P., Saccon, D., & Favaro, A. (1997). Burden and psychiatric symptoms on key relatives of patients with eating disorders: A preliminary study. *Eating and Weight Disorders-Studies on Anorexia, Bulimia and Obesity*, *2*(1), 44–48.

Schmidt, U., Lee, S., Beecham, J., Perkins, S., Treasure, J., Yi, I., . . . Johnson-Sabine, E. (2007). A randomized controlled trial of family therapy and cognitive behavior therapy guided self-care for adolescents with bulimia nervosa and related disorders. *American Journal of Psychiatry*, *164*(4), 591–598.

Sepulveda, A. R., Todd, G., Whitaker, W., Grover, M., Stahl, D., & Treasure, J. (2010). Expressed emotion in relatives of patients with eating disorders following skills training program. *International Journal of Eating Disorders*, *43*(7), 603–610.

Simic, M., Anderson, L. K., Berner, L., Peck, S. K., Hunt, K., Kaye, W., & Eisler, I. (2016). When family therapy isn't enough: New treatment directions for highly anxious and Dysregulated adolescents with anorexia nervosa. In S. B. Murray, L. K. Anderson, & L. Cohn (Eds.), *Innovations in family therapy for eating disorders: Novel treatment developments, patient insights, and the role of Carers*. New York: Routledge.

Szmukler, G. I., Berkowitz, R., Eisler, I., Leff, J., & Dare, C. (1987). "Expressed emotion" in individual and family settings: A comparative study. *British Journal of Psychiatry*, *151*, 174–178.

Szmukler, G. I., Eisler, I., Russell, G. F. M., & Dare, C. (1985). Parental "expressed emotion", anorexia nervosa and dropping out of treatment. *British Journal of Psychiatry*, *147*, 265–271.

Treasure, J., & Schmidt, U. (2013). The cognitive-interpersonal maintenance model of anorexia nervosa revisited: A summary of the evidence for cognitive, socio-emotional and interpersonal predisposing and perpetuating factors. *Journal of Eating Disorders*, *1*(1), 13.

Uehara, T., Kawashima, Y., Goto, M., Tasaki, S. I., & Someya, T. (2001). Psychoeducation for the families of patients with eating disorders and changes in expressed emotion: A preliminary study. *Comprehensive Psychiatry*, *42*(2), 132–138.

van Furth, E. F., van Strien, D. C., Martina, L. M., van Son, M. J., Hendrickx, J. J., & van Engeland, H. (1996). Expressed emotion and the prediction of outcome in adolescent eating disorders. *International Journal of Eating Disorders*, *20*(1), 19–31.

van Furth, E. F., van Strien, D. C., van Son, M. J., & Van Engeland, H. (1993). The validity of the five-minute speech sample as an index of expressed emotion in parents of eating disorder patients. *Journal of Child Psychology and Psychiatry*, *34*(7), 1253–1260.

Van Humbeeck, G., Van Audenhove, C., De Hert, M., Pieters, G., & Storms, G. (2002). Expressed emotion: A review of assessment instruments. *Clinical Psychology Review*, *22*(3), 321–341.

Vaughn, C. E. (1989). Expressed emotion in family relationships. *Child Psychology & Psychiatry & Allied Disciplines*, *30*(1), 13–22.

Vaughn, C. E., & Leff, J. (1976). The measurement of expressed emotion in the families of psychiatric patients. *British Journal of Social and Clinical Psychology*, *15*(2), 157–165.
Wager, T. D., & Ochsner, K. N. (2005). Sex differences in the emotional brain. *Neuroreport*, *16*(2), 85–87.
Wallis, A., Rhodes, P., Dawson, L., Miskovic-Wheatley, J., Madden, S., & Touyz, S. (2017). Relational containment: Exploring the effect of family-based treatment for anorexia on familial relationships. *Journal of Eating Disorders*, *5*(1), 27.
Watson, H. J., Yilmaz, Z., Thornton, L. M., Hübel, C., Coleman, J. R., Gaspar, H. A., . . . Bulik, C. M. (2019). Genome-wide association study identifies eight risk loci and implicates metabo-psychiatric origins for anorexia nervosa. *Nature Genetics*, *51*, 1207–1214.
Whitney, J., & Eisler, I. (2005). Theoretical and empirical models around caring for someone with an eating disorder: The reorganization of family life and inter-personal maintenance factors. *Journal of Mental Health*, *14*(6), 575–585.
Wiedemann, G., Rayki, O., Feinstein, E., & Hahlweg, K. (2002). The family questionnaire: Development and validation of a new self-report scale for assessing expressed emotion. *Psychiatry Research*, *109*(3), 265–279.

4

Assessment of Expressed Emotion

Erica Allan, Renee D. Rienecke, and Elizabeth K. Hughes

Introduction

Expressed emotion (EE) is a way of describing the characteristics of interpersonal interactions and the relationship between an individual with an illness or condition and their caregiver or other relative (Brown & Rutter, 1966; Hodes, Dare, Dodge, & Eisler, 1999; Vaughn & Leff, 1976a). Measurement of EE involves the assessment of the attitudes, emotions, and feelings expressed by a family member towards the relative with an illness (Rein et al., 2006) and reflects the extent to which critical, hostile, or emotionally overinvolved attitudes are expressed (Hooley & Parker, 2006). High-EE family members are generally characterized as being critical or hostile towards the unwell family member and/or emotionally overinvolved (Brown & Rutter, 1966; Rienecke, Accurso, Lock, & Le Grange, 2016).

EE has been found to be a consistent psychosocial predictor of treatment outcome and psychiatric relapse in a wide range of physical and psychological illnesses such as eating disorders, depression, anxiety, and substance abuse (Butzlaff & Hooley, 1998; Hooley & Parker, 2006; Rienecke et al., 2016). Specifically, research has demonstrated that patients living in high-EE family environments are at a significantly increased risk of early relapse across a number of psychiatric illnesses compared with patients who do not live in high-EE family environments (Butzlaff & Hooley, 1998; Hooley & Parker, 2006).

Several measures of EE are available, including semi-structured interviews, speech samples, and brief self-report questionnaires. Each of these varies considerably in the training and time required to administer and score. Further, the way in which EE is defined within these frameworks also varies. This chapter examines the methods of EE measurement, first focusing on interviewer-administered measures and then examining questionnaire-based measures.

Semi-Structured Interviews

Camberwell Family Interview

The Camberwell Family Interview (CFI) (Vaughn & Leff, 1976b) is a semi-structured interview used to measure EE. It has been referred to as the "gold standard" measure of EE (Hooley & Parker, 2006). Although it was originally developed within the context of schizophrenia (Vaughn & Leff, 1976a), it has been used extensively in research related to eating disorders (Hodes et al., 1999; Rein et al., 2006; Szmukler, Eisler, Russell, & Dare, 1985; van Furth, van Strien, van Son, & van Engeland, 1993).

The CFI is conducted with the relative of a patient on a one-on-one basis, with the respondent typically being the parent or spouse of the patient (Vaughn & Leff, 1976b). The duration of the interview can last from one to two hours in length and is recorded for later coding, which can take two to three hours. To be able to administer and score the CFI, between 40 and 88 hours, or approximately two weeks, of formal training must be completed (Duclos, Vibert, Mattar, & Godart, 2012).

Throughout the CFI, the interviewer seeks to obtain information about issues relating to the history of the patient's illness, including onset and symptoms, the impact of the illness on the family, arguments within the home, information regarding other problematic behaviors that the patient displays or engages in, the relationship between the relative and patient, and the relative's attitudes towards the illness (Vaughn & Leff, 1976a, 1976b).

Once administered and scored, the CFI provides an overall binary rating of EE as either high or low. Additionally, the CFI yields ratings on five subscales: Critical Comments, Hostility, Emotional Overinvolvement (EOI), Warmth, and Positive Remarks. The Critical Comments subscale reflects expression of resentment or disappointment, while Hostility reflects rejection of, or negative attitudes toward, the patient, particularly toward the patient as a person, rather than the patients' behaviors (Brown, Birley, & Wing, 1972; Vaughn & Leff, 1976b). The EOI subscale reflects distinct attitudes and behaviors of the relative that represent concern as manifested by overprotection, self-sacrifice, or heightened emotional reactivity (Brown et al., 1972; Vaughn & Leff, 1976b).

In regards to scoring, frequency counts are made for Critical Comments and Positive Remarks. Hostility is rated on a four-point scale from zero to three (absent, low, moderate, high), and is arrived at by considering the responses of the relative throughout the interview and whether there is evidence of criticism or rejection of the patient (Vaughn & Leff, 1976b). EOI is rated on a 6-point scale from 0 to 5 (absent to high). Ratings of EOI are made on the basis of reported overprotective or self-sacrificing behaviors of the parent or extreme emotional responses by the parent during the interview or towards the patient (e.g. crying during the interview) (Vaughn & Leff, 1976b). Warmth is rated on a 6-point scale from 0 to 5 (absent to high), and the rating is based on expressions of sympathy for and interest in the patient, as well as the tone of voice when talking about the patient. As with the EOI scores, higher Warmth scores are indicative of greater warmth. According to the CFI criteria, scoring above specified cut-offs for Critical Comments, Hostility, and/or EOI subscales results in classification of family members as high EE (Leff & Vaughn, 1985). Families who do not reach cut-off scores are classified as being low EE (Leff & Vaughn, 1985).

The CFI has been found to have considerable concurrent and predictive validity. For example, Brown et al. (1972) found that patients with a diagnosis of schizophrenia who were living in a high-EE home environment, as measured by the CFI, had double the baseline relapse rates 9 to 12 months after returning home from hospitalization compared with those who were not living in a high EE-home environment.

It is important to note that the recommended cut-off scores for rating a family member as high EE and predicting relapse in patients varies according to the illness. For example, the CFI was successfully used to predict relapse in patients with schizophrenia when any of the following criteria were used: (1) a score of 6 or more on Criticism, (2) a score of 3 or more on the EOI subscale, or (3) a score of more than 0 on Hostility (Vaughn & Leff, 1976a). In research on unipolar depression, two or three Critical Comments were found to be associated with poor outcome, whereas six Critical Comments were found to be necessary in the case of bipolar depression (Butzlaff & Hooley, 1998). Within the area of eating disorders, the cut-off scores for determining high EE based on Critical Comments varies among studies (Eisler et al., 2000; Szmukler, Berkowitz, Eisler, Leff, & Dare, 1987; Szmukler et al., 1985; van Furth et al., 1993), although it has been found that even low levels of Critical Comments are related to poor treatment outcome (Le Grange et al., 2011).

There are a number of problematic aspects to the administration and scoring of the CFI (Hooley & Parker, 2006). Foremost, the time and cost required to undergo comprehensive training in scoring and administration procedures could be prohibitive for many clinicians and researchers. Further, the duration of the CFI administration and subsequent coding and scoring of the interview could be troublesome for patients and examiners (Hooley & Parker, 2006; Magaña, Goldstein, Karno, & Miklowitz, 1986). In addition to these difficulties, the family member is required to be present for the face-to-face interview, which could prove difficult for some clinicians, researchers, and families. Thus, there have been efforts to develop briefer, but equally reliable, face-to-face measures of EE, such as the Standardized Clinical Family Interview (SCFI – Kinston & Loader, 1984) and Five-Minute Speech Sample (FMSS) (Magaña et al., 1986).

Standardized Clinical Family Interview

The Standardized Clinical Family Interview (SCFI) (Kinston & Loader, 1984) is a structured interview that was originally developed as a measure of general family interaction styles and subsequently adapted as a measure of EE and alternative to the CFI (Hodes et al., 1999). In contrast to the CFI, the SCFI is conducted with all family members as a group rather than just a parent or spouse. The duration of the interview is typically between 45 to 60 minutes and is audio or video recorded for subsequent rating. As part of the interview, the family is led by the interviewer in discussions and questioning related to the following topics: the way in which the family perceives itself, family cohesion, the way in which family members spend time together, similarities and differences between family members, the various roles and responsibilities within the household, discipline, conflict and conflict resolution, decision making, and family involvement with extended family and community (Kinston & Loader, 1984). Assessment of EE through the SCFI provides an overall EE rating and similar rating scales to the CFI, including Critical Comments, Positive Remarks, Hostility, EOI, and Warmth.

The SCFI has been used in eating disorder research (Eisler et al., 2000; Hoste & Le Grange, 2008; Le Grange, Eisler, Dare, & Hodes, 1992), but the criteria for classifying families as high EE have differed among studies. For example, the SCFI was used to assess EE in a treatment study of adolescents with anorexia nervosa (AN) (Le Grange et al., 1992) whereby highly critical families were defined as the presence of >2 Critical Comments made by the mother during the baseline SCFI, and low-EE families defined as the presence of <2 CCritical Comments made by the mother during the baseline SCFI. In contrast, Le Grange et al. (2011) and Rienecke et al. (2016) used the following criteria for rating high EE as measured by the SCFI: the presence of >1 Critical Comment, a rating of >1 for Hostility, or an EOI rating of >3. This further contrasts with studies of EE in schizophrenia, whereby high EE has typically been defined as >6 Critical Comments, a rating of >1 for Hostility, or an EOI rating of >3 (Vaughn & Leff, 1976a). These differences may be important to note in measuring EE in families of relatives with eating disorders, as it may reflect that these families typically express lower EE (Le Grange et al., 1992, 2011; van Furth et al., 1996), or that the threshold for assigning a rating of high EE needs to be adjusted as even low EE has been found to be related to treatment outcome in this population.

The SCFI has been reported to be a reliable measure for the assessment of family functioning (Kinston & Loader, 1986) and when used as a measure of EE has been reported to correlate well with the CFI (Hodes et al., 1999). In regard to interrater reliability, the Critical Comments subscale was found to have an interrater reliability of $\kappa = .76$, the Positive Remarks subscale was found to have an interrater reliability of $\kappa = .80$, Hostility $k = .71$, and Warmth $\kappa = .67$, and the EOI subscale was found to have an interrater reliability of $\kappa = .30$ (Hodes et al., 1999). Hodes et al. (1999) found a moderate correlation between the Critical Comments subscales of the CFI and SCFI $r_s = .531$, as well as the EOI subscales on the CFI and SCFI $r = .451$. A moderate correlation was found between the Warmth subscales on the CFI and SCFI $r = .508$, whereas a weak correlation between the Positive Remarks subscales on the CFI and SCFI was found r = .255 (Hodes et al., 1999). The CFI was found to elicit an increased level of Critical Comments when compared with the SCFI ($p = .035$).

Although the correlations between the SCFI and the CFI were found to be relatively low, this could be somewhat explained by the content of the CFI being more focused on symptomatic aspects of a patient's illness in comparison with the SCFI. The different focus of the interviews could result in differences in the content discussed within the SCFI and therefore may not provide the opportunity for respondents to elicit Critical Comments. Despite this, the significant reduction in time required to conduct the SCFI and the ability for it to be used as a general assessment of family interaction styles from which EE can also be rated makes the SCFI a reasonable alternative to the CFI. Although it must be considered that the training in administration and scoring as well as the time taken to conduct the SCFI with family members, while less than the CFI, may remain burdensome for some. The FMSS (Magaña et al., 1986) is a potential solution to the difficulty of requiring family members to participate in an extended assessment interview.

Five-Minute Speech Sample

The Five-Minute Speech Sample (FMSS) (Magaña et al., 1986) was developed as a brief measure of EE that can be used as an alternative to semi-structured or structured interviews, such as the CFI or SCFI. The FMSS is an interviewer-administered measure that is used to assess families of patients with a psychiatric illness. It is a five-minute interview in which the respondent, typically a family member, is asked to talk about the patient and their relationship; the interview is conducted individually, without the presence of other family members or the patient (Magaña et al., 1986). At the start of the interview, the following instructions are provided to the respondent: "I'd like to hear your thoughts about [name] in your own words and without my interrupting you with any questions or comments. When I ask you to begin, I'd like you to speak for five minutes, telling me what kind of a person [name] is and how the two of you get along together. After you have begun to speak, I prefer not to answer any questions. Are there any questions you would like to ask me before we begin?" (Magaña-Amato, 2012, p. 3). After these instructions have been provided to the respondent, the assessor does not give the respondent additional prompts, and the recording continues until the five minutes have lapsed (Magaña et al., 1986). The interview is audio recorded for later coding using a standardized system (Magaña-Amato, 2012). In contrast to the lengthy administration and coding of the CFI and SCFI, the FMSS requires five minutes to conduct and 20 minutes to code.

Assessment of EE using the FMSS includes rating the respondent's Initial Statement, Relationship, Criticism, Dissatisfaction, and EOI. The dimensions of Criticism, Relationship, and Emotional Overinvolvement are used to determine a high EE rating (Magaña et al., 1986). One or more critical comments, a negative relationship rating, a critical statement at the beginning of the interview, or a combination of those results in a high Criticism rating and subsequent overall high EE rating (Magaña et al., 1986). The EOI subscale is rated as high if there is either or both an emotional display during the interview (e.g. crying), evidence of excessive emotional involvement as reflected in self-sacrificing or overprotective behavior, and any two of the following: the respondent providing excessive detail about the relative that is related to the past, one or more statements of attitude (e.g. expressions of love), and excessive praise (five or more Positive Remarks made by the respondent about the relative).

A high EE classification is made if either or both high Criticism or high EOI is scored. In contrast to the CFI and SCFI, the FMSS does not contain measures of Hostility or Warmth. However, Hostility is frequently highly correlated with Criticism and is rarely present in the absence of Criticism or Critical Comments (Van Humbeeck, Van Audenhove, De Hert, Pieters, & Storms, 2002; Wearden, Tarrier, Barrowclough, Zastowny, & Rahill, 2000), which may explain the absence of its inclusion in the FMSS.

Ratings of EE derived from the FMSS have been demonstrated to have a reasonable degree of correspondence to those obtained by the CFI (Magaña et al., 1986). Magaña et al. (1986) examined the FMSS in relation to the CFI and found a high degree of correspondence between ratings of high EE on both the FMSS and CFI ($\chi 2 = 11.429, p < .001$). In addition, when a relative was identified as high EE, the subtype (Criticism or EOI) observed was similar for the FMSS and CFI ($\chi 2 = 8.04$, *df* = 1, $p < .005$). However, Magaña et al. (1986) also found that high EE was under-identified, with 20% of relatives rated as low EE on the FMSS and high EE on the CFI. This suggests that the FMSS may be less likely to elicit Critical Comments or EOI, or both, than the CFI.

Further evidence for the validity of the FMSS as a measure of EE comes from Rein et al. (2006), who examined the FMSS in relation to the CFI by conducting a study comparing EE ratings as measured by the FMSS with those obtained by the CFI. Participants included 40 parents from 22 families of adolescents with AN with an average age of 15.55 years (SD = 1.65). Participants were interviewed according to the protocol of each measure. The study found that ratings of overall EE and EOI obtained using the FMSS were significantly related to those measured by the CFI. Further, the FMSS was found to be a reliable measure of EE in reference to the CFI in terms of overall EE rating and EOI.

The FMSS has been widely used in eating disorder research settings (Le Grange et al., 2016; Rein et al., 2006; van Furth et al., 1993) and has been found to be a reliable measure of EE, with overall EE and EOI on the FMSS found to be significantly correlated with the corresponding ratings on the CFI (Rein et al., 2006).

As a measure of EE, the FMSS can be considered advantageous over the CFI or SCFI because it does not require formal training for researchers or clinicians to begin administration. In addition, the training and time required for administration and coding are significantly less than those for the CFI or SCFI. However, the training required for coding is substantial, taking approximately one week. Further, the duration of scoring required for each speech sample can be 20 minutes per sample (Magaña et al., 1986). Several questionnaire measures have been developed as a way of addressing the need to reduce training and administration time, which are discussed next.

Self-Report Scales and Questionnaires

Although semi-structured interviews and speech samples have been widely researched and used extensively within clinical research settings and provide a rich source of information on family interactions and relationships, there are several difficulties associated with their use. As mentioned, the CFI and SCFI require extensive training to administer and score them. Additionally, the CFI, SCFI, and FMSS require a face-to-face interview with family members of the unwell relative, which may be prohibitive in the assessment of EE. The FMSS is advantageous in that it does not require extensive training before it can be administered, but it does require training to score it. As a result, several self-report questionnaires have been developed to enable researchers and clinicians to reliably evaluate EE in relatives and patients without having to engage families and patients with lengthy interviews or commit to extensive training.

Level of Expressed Emotion Scale

The Level of Expressed Emotion (LEE) Scale (Cole & Kazarian, 1988) is a 60-item questionnaire that assesses the perceived EE of an important person in an unwell person's life over the past three months. Typically, the LEE is used to assess the EE of the relative or spouse from the point of view of the unwell person (i.e. the respondent is the unwell person), although a version of the LEE is also available for the relative to complete, in which the relative is required to evaluate their relationship with the unwell individual (Cole & Kazarian, 1988). The LEE is reported to require between 10 and 15 minutes to administer and score.

Items within the LEE are based on the EE construct as described and measured by Vaughn and Leff (1976a) and include the following four subscales: Intrusiveness, Negative Attitude, Tolerance and Expectations, and Emotional Response. There are 15 items within each subscale, with each item presented in a true/false response format. The LEE provides an overall EE score as well as a score for each of the four subscales. Once scored, the items on the LEE generate a score ranging from 60 to 120, with greater scores indicating a higher level of EE. The suggested procedure for classifying a score as high or low is to calculate a median score for the total sample, with scores above the median labeled as high and scores below the median labeled as low (Cole & Kazarian, 1993).

The LEE was reported to have high internal consistency for the total scale and subscales (Cole & Kazarian, 1988) and was reported to have demonstrated high test–retest reliability among a population of patients diagnosed with schizophrenia (r =.82, p <.01) (Cole & Kazarian, 1988). However, only a moderate correlation of r =.32 was found between the total LEE score on the patient version and the number of Critical

Comments made by a relative during the CFI, and a moderate correlation of r =.38 between the Critical Comments made by a relative during the CFI and the total score on the LEE relative version was found (Kazarian, Malla, Baker, & Cole, 1990). The patient version of the LEE was reported by Cole and Kazarian (1993) to be a good predictor of relapse in patients diagnosed with schizophrenia, with readmission rates found to be higher at two and five years post-discharge among those who obtained high LEE scores upon their initial admission and assessment compared with those who did not obtain high LEE scores.

The LEE has been used in research examining perceived EE in patients with eating disorders (Di Paola, Faravelli, & Ricca, 2010), and it is important to note that differing versions of the LEE are available and have been used in eating disorders research. The LEE, as developed by Cole and Kazarian (1988), was altered from its original format by Gerlsma, van der Lubbe, and van Nieuwenhuizen (1992), whereby the true/false response format was replaced with a 4-point Likert scale. Further, a principal-component analysis conducted by Gerlsma et al. (1992) reduced the number of items from 60 to 33, with three factors identified (Lack of Emotional Support, Intrusiveness/Control, and Irritability). Additionally, the LEE underwent further changes, with the addition of a Criticism subscale, which resulted in a 38-item measure of EE (Gerlsma & Hale, 1997), which was later used in research conducted by Moulds et al. (2000), whereby perceived EE was examined in a sample of women diagnosed with AN.

The LEE could be considered advantageous as a measure of EE in comparison with interview-based assessments such as the CFI, SCFI, or FMSS, as it does not require training in order to administer and score. Further, it requires significantly less time to administer than interview-based assessments of EE, requiring just 10–15 minutes. However, some considerations need to be taken into account when evaluating the LEE as a measure of EE. Primarily, the LEE was designed to measure *perceived* EE rather than serve as a direct observed measure of EE, and therefore the LEE could be considered as an alternative method to assess EE compared with the traditional measures (i.e. CFI, SCFI, FMSS). It could also be argued that perceived EE is a different construct altogether than observed EE. Thus, a self-report measure that assesses relative-reported

EE (i.e. from the perspective of the relative of the unwell patient) may also be required for comparison. The use of a measure of patient-reported perceived EE could also be problematic in a clinical population, as the perceptions of EE could be influenced by the symptoms of the respondent's illness, particularly in an ego-syntonic illness such as AN.

The Family Questionnaire

The Family Questionnaire (FQ) (Wiedemann, Rayki, Feinstein, & Hahlweg, 2002) is a 20-item questionnaire that was developed as a written questionnaire measure of EE. It was developed as an alternative measure to the CFI and can be administered without the need for extensive training in administration and scoring procedures, as well as significantly reduced administration and scoring time (Wiedemann et al., 2002). In completing the questionnaire, respondents are required to rate items that indicate how frequently they have responded in different ways to difficulties with their unwell family member. Examples of items include "I regard my own needs as less important", "It's hard for us to agree on things", "He/she irritates me", and "He/she is an important part of my life" (Wiedemann et al., 2002). Respondents rate items based on how frequently they have reacted to the unwell family member in that way (Never/Very Rarely = 1, Rarely = 2, Often = 3, Very Often = 4). There are two subscales within the FQ, EOI and Criticism, with each subscale containing ten items. The EOI subscale is designed to assess overconcern, overidentification, and overprotectiveness, whereas the Criticism subscale assesses critical attitudes and critical comments about the unwell family member. A score of 23 or higher on the Criticism subscale or 27 for EOI is recommended as the cut-off point for rating a respondent as high EE (Wiedemann et al., 2002).

The FQ was developed and tested using participants who were relatives of inpatients diagnosed with schizophrenia (Wiedemann et al., 2002). To be included in the study, patients were required to be living within the household of the relative or partner or have spent a minimum of ten hours per week with the relative or partner prior to their hospital admission. Two samples were used to develop the FQ; the first sample was composed of 76 relatives of 49 patients; the second sample was composed of 79 relatives of 50 patients and was used for the purposes of validation of the measure. The FQ initially comprised 130 items and was administered to the first sample for the purpose of item analysis. Thirty items that were highly correlated with the EOI and Criticism subscales of the CFI were selected for use in administration to the second sample and then further reduced to 20 items. EE ratings were obtained from participants within the second sample using the CFI and the FQ items. During the CFI, patterns of behavior in the three months leading up to the hospitalization were discussed, and the feelings towards and attitudes about the behaviors were observed, with six or more CCs resulting in a rating of high EE. Further, a rating of three or higher on the global index of EOI resulted in a rating of high EE.

The FQ has been reported to have good internal consistency for both the EOI subscale (ranging from 0.78 to 0.80) and the Critical Comments subscale (ranging from 0.91 to 0.92) (Wiedemann et al., 2002). Both subscales, as well as the total rating of EE, were found to correlate significantly with the CFI (Wiedemann et al., 2002). Specifically, the FQ was found to correctly identify the EE rating in 74% of respondents as classified by the CFI ($\chi 2 = 13.6$, $df = 1$, $p < .001$) (Wiedemann et al., 2002).

Although developed within a population of patients diagnosed with schizophrenia, the FQ has been used in research relating to AN. One such study (Moskovich, Timko, Honeycutt, Zucker, & Merwin, 2017) used the FQ to examine change in EE throughout the course of treatment for adolescents with AN. Additionally, the FQ has been used to examine EE in relation to carers of patients with AN in comparison with control families, with higher levels of EOI and Critical Comments found in the carers group (Kyriacou, Treasure, & Schmidt, 2008).

Little training is required for administration and scoring of the FQ, making it an accessible measure of EE. However, it is important to consider that the FQ provides a measure of EE through Critical Comments and EOI rather than encompassing the five aspects of EE as it was originally conceived. To assess EE in a comprehensive manner, employing the use of a broader measure of EE may be considered.

Additional Measures

There are several other written questionnaire measures of EE that have been developed over time. These measures are less-widely used or have limited psychometric data, so are briefly described here.

The Brief Dyadic Scale of Expressed Emotion (BDSEE) is a 14-item self-report measure designed to assess patients' perceptions of caregiver EE (Medina-Pradas, Navarro, López, Grau, & Obiols, 2011). It consists of three subscales: perceived criticism (e.g. "How disapproving is [caregiver] of what you do?"), perceived emotional overinvolvement (e.g. "[Caregiver] does not let me do things on my own"), and perceived warmth (e.g. "Do you feel loved by [caregiver]?"). Each answer is scored on a 10-point Likert scale (e.g. Never to Always, or Not at All Critical to Very Critical Indeed).

Although originally developed for relatives of patients with schizophrenia, Medina-Pradas and colleagues (2011) assessed the psychometric properties of the BDSEE with a sample of 77 adult patients with a diagnosis of an eating disorder (mean age 26.4, SD = 7.3, range 13–50) and their key relative. Correlations between patients' perceptions on the BDSEE and the objective ratings of the CFI were significant for CC ($r = 0.31$) and EOI ($r = 0.37$) but were not significant for Warmth ($r = 0.18$). The three BDSEE subscales were also significantly correlated with EE status (high versus low) as measured by the CFI (Criticism: $r = 0.40$; EOI: $r = 0.44$; Warmth: $r = -0.27$).

The Family Emotional Involvement and Criticism Scale (FEICS) is a 14-item self-report measure of perceived criticism and the intensity of emotional overinvolvement, also assessed from the patients' perspective (Shields, Franks, Harp, McDaniel, & Campbell, 1992). Items such as "My family knows what I am thinking before I tell them" and "My family approves of most everything I do" are measured on a 5-point Likert scale from Almost Never to Almost Always. The questionnaire was developed as part of a study examining family factors and cardiovascular health, so it was not designed with a specific psychiatric illness in mind, as with several other EE measures. Eighty-three patients with an average age of 55.5 years completed the measure. The authors found that perceived criticism was negatively correlated with family cohesion and adaptability, while EOI was positively correlated with cohesion and adaptability. The FEICS was not compared with EE as measured by the CFI or another objectively rated EE measure.

The Family Attitude Scale (FAS) is a written questionnaire that can be administered to the patient or to the patient's relative and is designed to assess EE (Kavanagh et al., 1997). The FAS is reported to require between 5 and 10 minutes to complete. It consists of 30 statements that describe an attitude or difficulty regarding the patient and requires the respondent to report on how often each statement has been true (Never = 0, Very Rarely = 1, Some Days = 2, Most Days = 3, Every Day = 4). Items within the FAS are designed to measure Criticism and Hostility and do not assess the other aspects of EE such as Warmth, EOI, and Positive Remarks. Example items include "He is really hard to take", "I feel very close to him" (reversed), "I argue with him", and "It is good to have him around" (reversed). Responses to the statement are tallied and provide a score between 0 and 120, with higher scores indicating higher levels of EE. Clinical and non-clinical normative data are available (Kavanagh et al., 1997).

The measure was developed using a sample of 228 undergraduate psychology students (65 male, 163 female) and their parents (137 mothers and 119 fathers), with data obtained from students and both parents in 112 cases (Kavanagh et al., 1997). The mean age of the students was 19.5 years, and the majority of students were born in Australia (81%) and spoke English as their first language (86%). Of the 228 students, 83% were living with one or both parents.

In a comparison between the FAS and the CFI in a clinical population, Kavanagh et al. (1997) administered both the CFI and FAS to 70 inpatients (46 males, 24 females) diagnosed with schizophrenia and found the total FAS scores to be significantly correlated with Criticism as measured by the CFI ($r = .38$, $p < .001$ for fathers; $r = .66$, $p < .01$ for mothers). Additionally, total FAS scores were significantly correlated with Hostility ratings made from the CFI ($r = .31$, $p < .05$ for fathers; $r = .39$, $p < .01$ for mothers). Using a FAS cut-off score of >50, it was determined that the FAS was able to successfully identify 71% of the high-EE families (based on Criticism) and 62% of the low-EE families (based on Criticism) that were identified by the CFI.

Moulds et al. (2000) examined the FAS in relation to the LEE and found a correlation of $r = .53$ between patients' ratings of siblings on the perceived criticism scale of the LEE and sibling self-report as measured by the FAS. However, this correlation was not significant, albeit due to low power given the small sample size ($n = 12$).

Overall, the FAS is a potentially suitable measure of EE, particularly when an efficient measure that has validity with regard to the CFI is required. The FAS also appears to be a good measure of EE in regards to the Hostility and Criticism aspect of EE. However, one of the disadvantages of the FAS is that it measures Criticism and Hostility only and does not measure the other aspects of EE, such as Warmth, EOI, or Positive Remarks. This could explain why the FAS has not been widely used as a measure of EE in populations with eating disorders, and therefore more research into the applicability of the FAS in this population may be required.

Conclusion

Numerous measures of EE are available, and they all present with advantages and disadvantages. The CFI (Vaughn & Leff, 1976b) is a reliable measure that has been used extensively in clinical and research settings. However, there are several disadvantages, including the level of training and time required to administer and code. The SCFI (Kinston & Loader, 1984) presents a useful alternative to the CFI but still requires investment in training and is generally not highly correlated with the CFI. The FMSS (Magaña et al., 1986) is advantageous in that it does not require training to administer but requires training to code. Further, it appears to not be as sensitive in identifying high EE as the CFI. Self-report questionnaire measures of EE are advantageous in that they can be completed relatively efficiently and without the need for face-to-face interviewing or substantial investment in training. However, there may be important differences in the constructs measured using questionnaires compared with interviews. For example, the LEE (Cole & Kazarian, 1988) is a measure of perceived EE as reported by the patient rather than EE as observed by an interviewer. Although this has its advantages in some areas of research and clinical practice, it could be highly influenced by patient symptoms and perceptions. Similarly, the FEICS (Shields et al., 1992) and BDSEE (Medina-Pradas et al., 2011) also measure perceived EE and include similar disadvantages to the LEE. The FAS is primarily a measure of Criticism and Hostility rather than a measure of the broader concept of EE. While this may be useful in settings in which there is a focus on Criticism and Hostility, it does not provide a complete measure of EE. Similarly, the FQ measures two aspects of EE, which is highly advantageous when an efficient measure of Criticism and EOI is required but not when a broader understanding of EE is required. When deciding on a measure of EE, consideration should be given to the setting in which EE will be measured; the frequency of administration; the availability of time and resources for training, administration, and scoring; and the purpose of obtaining the EE rating, including which ratings are of most interest.

References

Brown, G. W., Birley, J. L., & Wing, J. K. (1972). Influence of family life on the course of schizophrenic disorders: A replication. *British Journal of Psychiatry*, *121*(562), 241–258. doi:10.1192/bjp.121.3.241

Brown, G. W., & Rutter, M. (1966). The measurement of family activities and relationships: A methodological study. *Human Relations*, *19*(3), 241–263. doi:10.1177/001872676601900301

Butzlaff, R. L., & Hooley, J. M. (1998). Expressed emotion and psychiatric relapse: A meta-analysis. *Archives of General Psychiatry*, *55*(6), 547–552. doi:10.1001/archpsyc.55.6.547

Cole, J. D., & Kazarian, S. S. (1988). The level of expressed emotion scale: A new measure of expressed emotion. *Journal of Clinical Psychology*, *44*(3), 392–397. doi:10.1002/1097-4679(198805)44:3<392::AID-JCLP2270440313>3.0.CO;2-3

Cole, J. D., & Kazarian, S. S. (1993). Predictive validity of the Level of Expressed Emotion (LEE) scale: Readmission follow-up data for 1, 2, and 5-year periods. *Journal of Clinical Psychology*, *49*(2), 216–218. doi:10.1002/1097-4679(199303)49:2<216::AID-JCLP2270490214>3.0.CO;2-G

Di Paola, F., Faravelli, C., & Ricca, V. (2010). Perceived expressed emotion in anorexia nervosa, bulimia nervosa, and binge-eating disorder. *Comprehensive Psychiatry*, *51*(4), 401–405. doi:10.1016/j.comppsych.2009.10.002

Duclos, J., Vibert, S., Mattar, L., & Godart, N. (2012). Expressed emotion in families of patients with eating disorders: A review of the literature. *Current Psychiatry Reviews*, *8*(3), 183–202. doi:10.2174/157340012800792975

Eisler, I., Dare, C., Hodes, M., Russell, G., Dodge, E., & Le Grange, D. (2000). Family therapy for adolescent anorexia nervosa: The results of a controlled comparison of two family interventions. *Journal of Child Psychology and Psychiatry*, *41*(6), 727–736. doi:10.1111/1469-7610.00660

Gerlsma, C., & Hale, W. W. (1997). Predictive power and construct validity of the Level of Expressed Emotion (LEE) scale: Depressed out-patients and couples from the general community. *British Journal of Psychiatry*, *170*(6), 520–525. doi:10.1192/bjp.170.6.520

Gerlsma, C., van der Lubbe, P. M., & van Nieuwenhuizen, C. (1992). Factor analysis of the Level of Expressed Emotion scale: A questionnaire intended to measure "perceived expressed emotion". *British Journal of Psychiatry*, *160*(3), 385–389. doi:10.1192/bjp.160.3.385

Hodes, M., Dare, C., Dodge, E., & Eisler, I. (1999). The assessment of expressed emotion in a standardised family interview. *Journal of Child Psychology and Psychiatry*, *40*(4), 617–625. doi:10.1111/1469-7610.00478

Hooley, J. M., & Parker, H. A. (2006). Measuring expressed emotion: An evaluation of the shortcuts. *Journal of Family Psychology*, *20*(3), 386–396. doi:10.1037/0893-3200.20.3.386

Hoste, R. R., & Le Grange, D. (2008). Expressed emotion among white and ethnic minority families of adolescents with bulimia nervosa. *European Eating Disorders Review*, *16*(5), 395–400. doi:10.1002/erv.856

Kavanagh, D. J., O'Halloran, P., Manicavasagar, V., Clark, D., Piatkowska, O., Tennant, C., & Rosen, A. (1997). The family attitude scale: Reliability and validity of a new scale for measuring the emotional climate of families. *Psychiatry Research*, *70*(3), 185–195. doi:10.1016/S0165-1781(97)00033-4

Kazarian, S. S., Malla, A. K., Baker, B., & Cole, J. D. (1990). Comparisons of two expressed emotion scales with the Camberwell family interview. *Journal of Clinical Psychology*, *46*(3), 306–309. doi:10.1002/1097-4679(199005)46:3<306::AID-JCLP2270460310>3.0.CO;2-2

Kinston, W., & Loader, P. (1984). Eliciting whole-family interaction with a standardized clinical interview. *Journal of Family Therapy*, *6*(3), 347–363. doi:10.1046/j.1467-6427.1984.00655.x

Kinston, W., & Loader, P. (1986). Preliminary psychometric evaluation of a standardized clinical family interview. *Journal of Family Therapy*, *8*(4), 351–369. doi:10.1046/j.1986.00731.x

Kyriacou, O., Treasure, J., & Schmidt, U. (2008). Expressed emotion in eating disorders assessed via self-report: An examination of factors associated with expressed emotion in carers of people with anorexia nervosa in comparison to control families. *International Journal of Eating Disorders*, *41*(1), 37–46. doi:10.1002/eat.20469

Leff, J., & Vaughn, C. E. (1985). *Expressed emotion in families: Its significance for mental illness*. New York: Guilford Press.

Le Grange, D., Eisler, I., Dare, C., & Hodes, M. (1992). Family criticism and self-starvation: A study of expressed emotion. *Journal of Family Therapy*, *14*(2), 177–192. doi:10.1046/j.1992.00451.x

Le Grange, D., Hoste, R. R., Lock, J., & Bryson, S. W. (2011). Parental expressed emotion of adolescents with anorexia nervosa: Outcome in family-based treatment. *International Journal of Eating Disorders*, *44*(8), 731–734. doi:10.1002/eat.20877

Le Grange, D., Hughes, E. K., Court, A., Yeo, M., Crosby, R. D., & Sawyer, S. M. (2016). Randomized clinical trial of parent-focused treatment and family-based treatment for adolescent anorexia nervosa. *Journal of the American Academy of Child & Adolescent Psychiatry*, *55*(8), 683–692. doi:10.1016/j.jaac.2016.05.007

Magaña, A. B., Goldstein, M. J., Karno, M., & Miklowitz, D. J. (1986). A brief method for assessing expressed emotion in relatives of psychiatric patients. *Psychiatry Research*, *17*(3), 203–212. doi:10.1016/0165-1781(86)90049-1

Magaña-Amato, A. (2012). *Manual for coding expressed emotion from the five minute speech sample*. Los Angeles: UCLA Family Project.

Medina-Pradas, C., Navarro, J. B., López, S. R., Grau, A., & Obiols, J. E. (2011). Further development of a scale of perceived expressed emotion and its evaluation in a sample of patients with eating disorders. *Psychiatry Research*, *190*(2), 291–296. doi:10.1016/j.psychres.2011.06.011

Moskovich, A. A., Timko, C. A., Honeycutt, L. K., Zucker, N. L., & Merwin, R. M. (2017). Change in expressed emotion and treatment outcome in adolescent anorexia nervosa. *Eating Disorders: The Journal of Treatment & Prevention*, *25*(1), 80–91. doi:10.1080/10640266.2016.1255111

Moulds, M. L., Touyz, S. W., Schotte, D., Beumont, P. J. V., Griffiths, R., Russell, J., & Charles, M. (2000). Perceived expressed emotion in the siblings and parents of hospitalized patients with anorexia nervosa. *International Journal of Eating Disorders, 27*(3), 288–296. doi:10.1002/(SICI)1098-108X(200004)27:3<288::AID-EAT5>3.0.CO;2-7

Rein, Z., Perdereau, F., Curt, F., Jeammet, P., Fermanian, J., & Godart, N. (2006). Expressed emotion and anorexia nervosa: The validation of the five-minute speech sample in reference to the Camberwell family interview. *International Journal of Eating Disorders, 39*(3), 217–223. doi:10.1002/eat.20245

Rienecke, R. D., Accurso, E. C., Lock, J., & Le Grange, D. (2016). Expressed emotion, family functioning, and treatment outcome for adolescents with anorexia nervosa. *European Eating Disorders Review, 24*(1), 43–51. doi:10.1002/erv.2389

Shields, C. G., Franks, P., Harp, J. J., McDaniel, S. H., & Campbell, T. L. (1992). Development of the Family Emotional Involvement and Criticism Scale (FEICS): A self-report scale to measure expressed emotion. *Journal of Marital and Family Therapy, 18*, 395–407. doi:10.1111/j.1752-0606.1992.tb00953.x

Szmukler, G. I., Berkowitz, R., Eisler, I., Leff, J., & Dare, C. (1987). Expressed emotion in individual and family settings: A comparative study. *The British Journal of Psychiatry, 151*(2), 174–178. doi:10.1192/bjp.151.2.174

Szmukler, G. I., Eisler, I., Russell, G. F., & Dare, C. (1985). Anorexia nervosa, parental "expressed emotion" and dropping out of treatment. *The British Journal of Psychiatry, 147*(3), 265–271. doi:10.1192/bjp.147.3.265

van Furth, E. F., van Strien, D. C., Martina, L. M. L., van Son, M. J. M., Hendrickx, J. J. P., & van Engeland, H. (1996). Expressed emotion and the prediction of outcome in adolescent eating disorders. *International Journal of Eating Disorders, 20*(1), 19–31. doi:10.1002/(SICI)1098-108X(199607)20:1<19::AID-EAT3>3.0.CO;2-7

van Furth, E. F., van Strien, D. C., van Son, M. J. M., & van Engeland, H. (1993). The validity of the five-minute speech sample as an index of expressed emotion in parents of eating disorder patients. *Journal of Child Psychology and Psychiatry, 34*(7), 1253–1260. doi:10.1111/j.1469-7610.1993.tb01786.x

Van Humbeeck, G., Van Audenhove, C., De Hert, M., Pieters, G., & Storms, G. (2002). Expressed emotion: A review of assessment instruments. *Clinical Psychology Review, 22*(3), 321–341. doi:10.1016/S0272-7358(01)00098-8

Vaughn, C., & Leff, J. (1976a). The influence of family and social factors on the course of psychiatric illness: A comparison of schizophrenic and depressed neurotic patients. *The British Journal of Psychiatry, 129*(2), 125–137. doi:10.1192/bjp.129.2.125

Vaughn, C., & Leff, J. (1976b). The measurement of expressed emotion in the families of psychiatric patients. *British Journal of Social and Clinical Psychology, 15*(2), 157–165. doi:10.1111/j.2044-8260.1976.tb00021.x

Wearden, A. J., Tarrier, N., Barrowclough, C., Zastowny, T. R., & Rahill, A. A. (2000). A review of expressed emotion research in health care. *Clinical Psychology Review, 20*(5), 633–666. doi:10.1016/S0272-7358(99)00008-2

Wiedemann, G., Rayki, O., Feinstein, E., & Hahlweg, K. (2002). The family questionnaire: Development and validation of a new self-report scale for assessing expressed emotion. *Psychiatry Research, 109*(3), 265–279. doi:10.1016/S0165-1781(02)00023-9

5

Expressed Emotion and Anorexia Nervosa

Sasha Gorrell and Daniel Le Grange

Introduction

Expressed emotion (EE) has long been studied for its important role in treatment outcome and relapse for a broad range of adult and pediatric illnesses (Butzlaff & Hooley, 1998; Wearden, Tarrier, Barrowclough, Zastowny, & Rahill, 2000), including eating disorders (e.g., Rienecke, 2018). Of all the recognized eating disorders, EE has most commonly been studied in patients with anorexia nervosa (AN) and to a lesser extent in patients with bulimia nervosa (BN). This chapter traces the origin of the study of EE in AN, along with a summary of research evidence regarding patient and caregiver characteristics associated with EE and their relation to AN treatment outcome. Some studies in this chapter include transdiagnostic samples; whenever possible, efforts to isolate findings specific to AN have been made. Throughout, clinical and theoretical implications are discussed, concluding with critical directions for future research.

Expressed Emotion and Treatment Outcome

Historical Beginnings

As family factors may play a non-specific role in the genesis and maintenance of AN (Le Grange, Lock, Loeb & Nicholls, 2010), relational constructs such as EE should naturally be included in the study of eating disorder treatment. When publication of studies addressing EE in the context of eating disorders originated in the mid 1980s, study of this construct among patients with schizophrenia and mood disorders had typically been conducted using the Camberwell Family Interview (CFI; Rutter & Brown, 1966; Vaughn & Leff, 1976). Considered a gold standard by which to measure EE, the CFI requires one to two hours to administer and is used to identify five components of EE among parents: (1) Critical Comments, (2) Hostility, (3) Emotional Overinvolvement (EOI), (4) Warmth, and (5) Positive Remarks (PR). While it is titled a "family interview", use of the CFI specifies that each parent be interviewed individually. In early study of families of patients with schizophrenia, parents were classified as "high EE" if either parent made six or more Critical Comments, scored three or above in EOI, or showed any Hostility (Leff & Vaughn, 1985; Vaughn & Leff, 1976). Lower cut-offs (i.e., two or three criticisms) have demonstrated validity in predicting clinical outcomes for families of patients with depression (Leff & Vaughn, 1985; Vaughn & Leff, 1976). In general, only a small number of families caring for patients with AN are characterized by high levels of Criticism and/or Hostility toward their offspring (e.g., Le Grange, Eisler, Dare, & Hodes, 1992; van Furth et al., 1996). For example, one recent study showed that fewer than a third (n = 32, 29%) of families of children with AN had at least one parent with high EE (Rienecke, Accurso, Lock, & Le Grange, 2016). Consequently, cut-offs for Critical Comments among families with AN have been lowered to as low as one (e.g., Le Grange, Hoste, Lock, & Bryson, 2011). Notably, for patients with AN, even a low level of criticism has been shown to negatively impact treatment outcomes (e.g., van Furth et al., 1996).

The first study to explore EE in AN treatment used a cut-off of six Critical Comments for mothers and three Critical Comments for fathers as criteria for high EE (Szmukler, Eisler, Russell, & Dare, 1985). This investigation specifically explored attrition in a sample of adolescents and adults receiving family or individual treatment for AN (n = 34) and BN (n = 17). In this study, determination of EE was made via the CFI, and ratings were established of the five EE components from audiotaped recordings. Across the full sample, results indicated increased attrition among patients with parents rated high in EE, i.e., when both fathers and mothers of patients who had dropped out of treatment demonstrated significantly elevated Critical Comments. Fathers, but not mothers, also demonstrated higher EOI in the dropout group (all *ps* $< .01$). Interactions were demonstrated relative to treatment type such that for family therapy, the strongest association was between mothers, elevated Critical Comments, and attrition ($p = .002$). For fathers, increased Critical Comments were more likely to be associated with attrition from individual supportive therapy ($p = .02$).

At the start of the next decade, Le Grange and colleagues (1992) attempted to further standardize the study of EE within adolescent eating disorder treatment. These authors departed from the individual-based CFI and instead opted to use the Standardized Clinical Family Interview (SCFI) (Kinston & Loader, 1984), which was purportedly more efficient and less subject to the vagaries of interviewer style and therapeutic setting (Le Grange et al., 1992). In an accompanying pilot treatment study ($N = 18$), the efficacy of conjoint family therapy was compared with a separated format of family therapy (i.e., individual supportive sessions for the patient and counseling for the parents) in a sample of adolescents with AN (Le Grange, Eisler, Dare, & Russell, 1992). Patients and their parents were interviewed together with the SCFI and video-recorded to code for EE specifically. While the pilot study was originally undertaken to discern the effective components of family therapy, results also revealed compelling between-group differences in EE. Specifically, findings indicated that parental criticism toward the unwell adolescent, if present at the beginning of therapy, rendered the therapy less effective. Patients of parents who were more critical at baseline were less likely to achieve "good" or "intermediate" outcomes according to the Morgan-Russell Scale ($p <.05$) (Morgan & Russell, 1975). After six months of therapy, Critical Comments ($p = .002$) and Hostility ($p <.05$) had risen significantly in the group that had done poorly, as compared with caregivers of those patients who had done better; Warmth was also significantly lower in this group ($p <.05$). Although there were no differences in EE scores between the two treatment groups at baseline, post-treatment levels of Critical Comments for those relatives who started out with elevated scores remained high. Likewise, parents who began treatment with lower levels of Critical Comments remained low. At the end of treatment, Critical Comments were at higher levels for parents participating in conjoint family therapy when compared with parents in the separated format. These findings suggest that high EE (based on Critical Comments) may experience a reduction in criticism of their child as more of a challenge in the context of conjoint family therapy.

Just a few years later, a study of Dutch families of adolescent patients with eating disorders ($N = 49$, 18 diagnosed with AN) used the CFI to evaluate EE, which the authors chose to consider as continuous, rather than dichotomous (i.e., high versus low EE) (van Furth et al., 1996). Study findings revealed that parental EE was low at baseline and decreased over the course of treatment. However, maternal criticism was the best predictor of poorer treatment outcome ($p < .01$), reflecting 34% of the variance in Morgan-Russell status at end of treatment and 28% at follow-up one year later. It should be noted, however, that this was a mixed diagnostic adolescent sample within which the maternal mean level of Critical Comments was significantly lower for patients with AN than those with eating disorder not otherwise specified (EDNOS) ($p < .05$).

Taken together, preliminary evidence across these first studies of EE in AN highlight the importance of noting elevated levels of EE, and in particular, the impact of Critical Comments on treatment outcomes. Generally, when parental criticism of the adolescent was high, families were more likely to drop out of treatment or have poor outcomes if they remained in treatment. Further, these initial studies hint that there may also be differences in the contribution of EE to treatment outcome relative to the gender of the parent or treatment type. While these studies should be interpreted with caution given their pilot sample nature, they laid important and notably consistent groundwork for future study of treatment outcome in this patient population.

Parental Criticism and Treatment Outcome: A Case for a Separated Format of Family Therapy?

As study of EE and adolescent eating disorder treatment has burgeoned, two comprehensive reviews have revealed a noted negative impact of high EE on AN treatment outcome among adolescents (c.f., Duclos, Vibert, Mattar, & Godart, 2012; Rienecke, 2018). While the type of EE that is implicated has varied across study samples, high EE has mostly been as a result of parental criticism rather than hostility or EOI. In a sample of adolescent patients with AN, Eisler and colleagues (2000) found that maternal criticism predicted poor treatment outcome, a finding that was still significant at five-year follow-up (Eisler, Simic, Russell, & Dare, 2007). In the initial study (Eisler et al., 2000), which followed the pilot study (Le Grange et al., 1992), adolescents with AN ($N = 40$) and their families were randomly assigned to either conjoint (CFT) or separated formats of family therapy (SFT); SFT consisted of individual supportive sessions for the patient and counseing sessions for the parents (Eisler et al., 2000). In this study, all patients demonstrated significant overall improvement (ps = .001), but the two forms of therapy did not demonstrate significant differences. However, for patients of families with high EE (i.e., maternal criticism), SFT trended toward superiority to CFT ($p = .05$). For all families, Critical Comments from parents to adolescents and between parents were significantly reduced (ps = .01). Over the course of treatment, all parents also demonstrated more warmth to one another ($p = .001$) but not to their child. While these results are relatively underpowered and only trended toward significance when comparing differences per treatment group, they aligned with prior preliminary findings demonstrated by Le Grange and colleagues (1992) that when parental criticism of the adolescent was high, families appeared to do better in separated rather than CFT.

At five-year follow-ups, there was a continued lack of significant differences between families with high versus low EE in most outcomes in this sample with the exception of two: history of inpatient treatment and having a critical mother (Eisler et al., 2007). Specifically, in the full sample, patients whose mothers had made three or more Critical Comments at baseline assessment were significantly more likely to have a "poor" outcome on the Morgan-Russell Scale at five-year follow-up ($p < .04$). Of note, the frequency of previous hospital admissions was nearly twice as high in the high EE group, but the difference between groups (i.e., high versus low EE) was not statistically significant. Patients from high-EE families had significantly lower baseline weight ($p < .04$), and when weight was entered into the model, associations between elevated baseline EE and outcome at five-year follow-ups were no longer statistically significant. Further, there was no association between end-of-treatment

EE and outcome at five-year follow-up. Despite the lack of significant differences in the full sample, moderation analyses indicated a significant interaction between treatment group, EE, and time. Specifically, those in the high-EE group treated with SFT continued to gain weight post-treatment, reaching an average of 99.9% of expected weight as compared with 85.8% in the CFT group (p <.04). In contrast, those in the low-EE group continued to gain weight at a similar rate (95%) compared with those in SFT (96.1%).

In secondary data analysis of a recent randomized control trial (RCT) that compared conjoint family-based treatment (FBT), a manualized version of the original family therapy utilized in the London studies, to a separated parent-focused treatment (PFT) for adolescents with AN (N = 107) (c.f., Le Grange et al., 2016), Allan, Le Grange, Sawyer, McLean, and Hughes (2018) examined associations between parental EE, remission, and illness severity and how EE may be impacted by the version of family treatment, conjoint or separated (Allan et al., 2018). Much like SFT, PFT is a separated form of FBT in which the adolescent meets with a nurse at the start of each session and only the parents meet with the clinician for therapy (Hughes, Sawyer, Loeb, & Le Grange, 2015). While all domains of EE were considered in this study, only high maternal criticism was related to longer duration of illness at baseline (p = .01). Contrary to a previous study (Eisler et al., 2000), there was no association found between high EE and lower pre-treatment weight.

Perhaps more important, findings indicated that treatment type was significantly associated with maternal criticism at the end of treatment, after controlling for both remission status, and baseline criticism (p = .01). Specifically, those randomized to PFT were more likely to evidence lower maternal criticism; with the noted covariates, these findings suggest that reductions in criticism were not simply a consequence of greater remission rates in PFT. As well, increases in maternal criticism were evidenced only for conjoint FBT and not in PFT (p = .001), consistent with the earlier work testing conjoint versus separated family therapy (Le Grange et al., 1992). In the full sample, adolescents of mothers who showed an increase, or remained high, in EE were less likely to remit compared with adolescents for whom EE decreased or remained low (p = 0.03); these findings were not indicated for paternal EE. In summary, these findings demonstrate that when parents, particularly mothers, were critical, patients did better in PFT. Further, high parental criticism is more likely to be reduced after PFT compared with FBT, regardless of treatment outcome.

In this work, we have noted the differences in EE and adolescent AN treatment outcome generally within conjoint versus separated family treatment formats (i.e., SFT or PFT). Departing from a comparison of different forms of family treatment, recent investigation has also examined the role of EE in impacting treatment outcomes in an RCT that compared the efficacy of FBT with an individual adolescent-focused therapy (AFT) in a sample of adolescents with AN (Lock et al., 2010; Rienecke et al., 2016). AFT is an individual psychotherapy focusing on enhancing self-efficacy, autonomy, individuation, and assertiveness while also including collateral parent meetings to support the adolescent in the treatment process (Fitzpatrick, Moye, Hoste, Lock, & Le Grange, 2010). In this RCT, baseline EE (measured via the SCFI) did not moderate end-of-treatment outcome or specifically predict remission (Le Grange et al., 2012). However, high maternal criticism was more likely to predict treatment dropout (p = .005) (Rienecke et al., 2016), mirroring the initial findings from Szmukler and colleagues (1985). Further, elevated paternal criticism at baseline was associated with less improvement in eating disorder pathology at the end of treatment (p = .0006). An interaction also emerged between maternal EE and treatment outcome, such that patients with mothers who demonstrated elevated hostility at baseline gained significantly more weight in the AFT group than those in the FBT group (p = .0002).

From historical beginnings, the reasonably consistent evidence that implicates high EE in the form of criticism, particularly maternal criticism, in poor treatment outcome leads one to speculate as to why this is the case. The differences between a conjoint format versus a separated format of family therapy center around the issue of being able to see the family as a whole or conjointly, as opposed to seeing parents separately from the adolescent with an eating disorder. Observation of transactional patterns in conjoint sessions is direct and allows the therapist to intervene in real time as the family is organizing itself around the abnormal behavior of their child. In contrast, in separated sessions, the therapist can only focus attention on how the caregivers may modify their behavior but does not allow for direct intervention on the more integrated family system. While preventing *in vivo* modification of interpersonal communication and while only speculative, working with the parents separately may serve to increase self-reflection, empathy for their child, and more constructive use of the session toward modifying caregiver behavior. One of the key tenets of FBT is to reduce parental criticism by way of externalizing the illness (Lock & Le Grange, 2013). What these studies seem to indicate is that, under circumstances in which criticism is elevated, this may be particularly well-achieved within the context of PFT rather than conjoint FBT.

Emotional Overinvolvement With Treatment Outcome

Domains of EE other than criticism (e.g., EOI) may also impact treatment outcome. A recent study investigated EE within an acceptance-based, separated form of FBT (ASFT) in a sample of adolescents with AN or sub-threshold AN ($N = 47$) and their families (Moskovich, Timko, Honeycutt, Zucker, & Merwin, 2017). In comparison with earlier work using a separated model of FBT (e.g., Eisler et al., 2000), the specific target of ASFT is increased psychological flexibility (i.e., capacity to experience difficult thoughts and feelings and to engage in effective and value-guided behavior), with emphasis on behavioral management and parental self-care (Moskovich et al., 2017). This study used the Family Questionnaire (FQ), completed by parents, which measures two facets of EE: Critical Comments and EOI (Wiedemann, Rayki, Feinstein, & Hahlweg, 2002). Findings indicated that parental EOI, but not Critical Comments, decreased after six months of treatment ($p < .05$). Further, change in maternal, but not paternal EE, were associated with lower eating disorder psychopathology at the end of treatment ($p < .05$). While these results should be interpreted conservatively, given a modest sample size and use of a self-report questionnaire (i.e., the FQ), they suggest that overinvolvement may diminish in a separated family therapy format and that this change in EE may be positively related to adolescent outcomes. Of note, while elevated EOI has consistently been implicated in the context of schizophrenia (Wearden et al., 2000), this is the only study to have found any evidence that this domain of EE singularly impacts treatment for adolescent AN.

Differences in Treatment Outcome Specific to Parent Gender

In contrast with studies that have found results only related to maternal EE, with no evidence that paternal EE may specifically impact treatment outcome (e.g., Allan et al., 2018), some work has identified findings specific to fathers. For example, in a study of adolescents and adults with AN or EDNOS-AN ($N = 177$), adolescent response to inpatient treatment was overall better than that for adults (Goddard, Hibbs, et al., 2013). In addition to other psychosocial features, perceived paternal control, defined as the psychological control displayed by the father toward the patient, and paternal EE were significantly related to eating disorder symptoms at discharge (ps $<.05$). Another recent study of adolescents receiving either FBT ($n = 55$) or PFT ($n = 51$) for adolescent AN investigated specific factors that were most likely to predict early response (i.e., early weight gain), as well as remission at end of treatment (Hughes, Sawyer, Accurso, Singh, & Le Grange, 2019). Results indicated that weight gain of 2.80 kg (FBT) or 2.27 kg (PFT) by session five was the best predictor of remission ($p = .004$), and low parental criticism was one of the significant predictors of this early response. Specifically, early response in FBT was predicted by factors including low paternal criticism ($p = .03$), whereas early response in PFT was predicted by factors including low maternal criticism ($p <.05$).

Differences in maternal versus paternal EE and treatment outcome were also found in another recent investigation of adolescent patients with AN receiving standard outpatient treatment or a systemic family therapy protocol ($N = 60$) (Duclos et al., 2018). In this study, when controlling for treatment group and baseline clinical status, high maternal EOI at baseline was significantly associated with lower eating disorder severity ($p = .02$), fewer re-hospitalizations ($p = .007$), and better nutritional status 18 months later ($p = .008$). No associations were found with paternal EE. This study has notable findings in that elevated EE, if in the form of maternal EOI, may actually play a positive role in AN. Given that these results appear to counter those of Goddard and colleagues (2013), in which EOI negatively contributed to treatment outcome, more research specific to the role of EOI is warranted.

Considering other domains of EE, only one study has specifically found isolated evidence of the impact of parental warmth on eating disorder treatment outcomes (Le Grange et al., 2011). These analyses evaluated patients with AN ($N = 86$) and their families who participated in an RCT comparing outcomes relative to two doses of FBT (short term versus longer term) for adolescent AN (Lock, Agras, Bryson, & Kraemer, 2005). For this study, EE was measured with the SCFI, and eating disorder outcomes were determined with Morgan-Russell scale ratings; families were categorized as high EE if either parent expressed any Critical Comments, any Hostility, or EOI >2. In this sample, ratings of Criticism and Hostility were low and similar for both parents, but mothers were more likely to exhibit EOI. Regarding treatment outcomes, there was no difference in the percent of families with high EE between the good versus poor outcome group ($p = .15$). However, patients with good outcomes were significantly more likely to have both mothers ($p = .01$) and fathers ($p = .04$) who exhibited Warmth. These findings underscore the potential importance of the positive domains of EE (i.e., Warmth and PR), which have been notably underrepresented in their connection with AN treatment outcome.

Parent and Patient Characteristics Associated With EE

Systematic review of caregiving in the broader context of eating disorders reveals that a majority of studies implicate high EE in negative outcomes, and most investigations have focused on samples of adolescents and maternal caregiving (Anastasiadou, Medina-Pradas, Sepulveda, & Treasure, 2014; Zabala, Macdonald, & Treasure, 2009). Within this extant literature, some studies have focused on specific patient and parent characteristics that are commonly associated with EE, including differences evidenced between maternal and paternal EE. Following early comparison of EE among families with schizophrenia and mood disorders (Vaughn & Leff, 1976), some research included the comparison of EE in these patient populations with those diagnosed with eating disorders (Butzlaff & Hooley, 1998) and medical diagnoses within broader health care (Wearden et al., 2000). In this path of inquiry, one study investigating differences between families of children with AN and those with cystic fibrosis found that families with AN demonstrated a greater proportion of parents with high EE than families of patients with cystic fibrosis; however, these differences were not significant (Blair, Freeman, &

Cull, 1995). Work specifically within the study of AN has identified patterns in correlates of EE specific to parent characteristics, including caregiver distress and burden, is detailed next.

Patterns in Correlates With EE

While levels of EE might be relatively low in families of children with AN, of parents who demonstrate high EE in the context of caregiving for a child with an eating disorder, patterns in EE may differ between parents. For example, in one of the first studies to include adolescent patients with AN, results revealed a moderately strong correlation between maternal criticism and EOI; this correlation was not evidenced among fathers (van Furth et al., 1996). Further, in this study, mothers who were critical of their offspring with an eating disorder were also more overinvolved, whereas in contrast, fathers were either critical *or* overinvolved. In a more recent study of inpatient and outpatient treatment for AN, the child's illness severity was associated with high EE and depression in parents ($p < .05$) (Schwarte et al., 2017). Specifically, mothers demonstrated higher EOI, Critical Comments, and depression scores than fathers (ps $< .05$). Duration of illness, intact family status, psychiatric comorbidity, and AN subtype did not significantly impact parental EE or depression. These findings are in contrast to those of Allan and colleagues (2018), who found that duration of illness, but not illness severity, was positively correlated with maternal criticism. Both the work of Schwarte and colleagues (2017) and Allan and colleagues (2018) consisted of secondary data analyses of RCT samples; the samples consisted of 102 or 172 adolescents with AN and their caregivers, respectively. Accordingly, it is possible that a discrepancy in findings between these two studies may be an artifact of comparative statistical power.

In an attempt to better understand parent and patient characteristics related to EE, one study ($N = 215$) compared EE among families of adolescents with major depressive disorder (i.e., psychiatric control group, $n = 40$), BN ($n = 54$), and AN ($n = 121$) (Rienecke et al., 2016). Results indicated that fathers demonstrated higher levels of Critical Comments toward patients with BN or major depressive disorder than those with AN, whereas mothers exhibited more Critical Comments toward patients with BN ($p = .003$) than those with depression or AN. Regardless of eating disorder diagnosis, the presence of siblings reduced both maternal warmth and EOI (*p*s = .004). Further, regarding family status, fathers from intact families demonstrated greater Warmth ($p = .04$) and fewer Critical Comments ($p < .001$) than fathers from nonintact families. In contrast, mothers from intact families were less critical ($p = .03$) but also made fewer Positive Remarks ($p = .04$) than mothers from nonintact families.

A study of patients with transdiagnostic eating disorders ($n = 79$) and their caregivers ($n = 126$) evaluated associations between parental psychopathology, EE, and patient symptom severity (Rienecke & Richmond, 2017). The majority of patients in this sample were diagnosed with AN ($n = 54$) or EDNOS-AN ($n = 18$). Findings indicated that mothers were more likely to be high EE as compared with fathers, expressing significantly more Critical Comments ($p = .01$) and EOI ($p < .001$) toward the unwell adolescent. Both mothers and fathers reported greater psychopathology compared with population norms ($p < .01$), and paternal psychopathology was positively related to EE. Maternal psychopathology was significantly related to total and subscale scores on adolescent eating pathology (*p*s <.01), and maternal criticism was significantly related to adolescent dietary restraint ($p = .006$); significant relations in these domains were not evidenced for fathers.

Only one study has investigated the potential association between EE and therapeutic alliance (Rienecke, Richmond, & Lebow, 2016). In this study, adolescents with AN and EDNOS-AN who were participating in a family-based partial hospitalization program ($n = 56$) and their caregivers ($n = 78$) reported on therapeutic alliance, EE, and associations with treatment outcome. Counter to hypotheses, findings indicated that EE was not associated with therapeutic alliance; however, maternal hostility did contribute to lower maternal alliance with the provider ($p = .05$).

In light of evidence that parental alliance and maternal hostility play critical roles in treatment outcome (Isserlin & Couturier, 2012; Le Grange et al.,1992), specific interventions aimed to decrease maternal hostility toward the patient might yield benefits for not only the alliance with the provider but also treatment outcome.

In summary, patterns in associations with EE among caregivers seem to implicate maternal criticism and EOI, as well as depression, over and above that of fathers. One exception may be the impact of paternal psychopathology on EE (Rienecke & Richmond, 2017). There also seems to be some advantage associated with intact family status in that it may yield greater paternal warmth and less criticism from both parents. Given these collective findings, it appears that parental psychopathology and hostility should be assessed in addition to EE at the beginning of treatment so that appropriate clinical interventions can be utilized. Regarding patient factors, results remain inconclusive regarding whether illness severity or duration of illness or their combination may be more related to parental EE toward their offspring with AN. These findings, as well as study of characteristics specific to patients that may interact with those of their respective caregivers, warrant future investigation.

Caregiver Burden and Distress

In recognition of the difficulty of caring for a loved one with a serious illness, several studies have specifically examined EE and its association with the experience of the caregiver. For example, one recent study of 50 mothers and 38 fathers of adolescents first hospitalized for AN treatment found that caregiving experience was significantly correlated with EE, as measured by the FQ (Blondin, Meilleur, Taddeo, & Frappier, 2019). Specifically, increased difficult behavior from the patient (e.g., patient acting moody, unpredictable) contributed to the most Critical Comments from both mothers ($p < .001$) and fathers ($p < .01$). Other studies have more comprehensively evaluated psychological distress, some with specific attention paid to caregiver burden. One study of 56 caregivers of adolescent and young adult patients with eating disorders, the majority of whom had AN ($n = 38$), evaluated associations between EE, measured with the FQ, and caregiver burden (Coomber & King, 2013). In this sample, caregivers demonstrated sustained and high levels of Critical Comments and EOI; significant decreases were noted in criticism from baseline (Time 1) to 4.5 months (Time 2) ($p < .01$), but no significant change was evidenced between Time 1 and 9 months (Time 3). EOI significantly decreased from Time 1 to Time 2 ($p < .01$), as well as from Time 1 to Time 3 ($p < .001$). Total EE was a significant, unique predictor of caregiver burden at Time 2 ($p < .05$).

In a sample of caregivers ($n = 97$) of adolescent patients with transdiagnostic eating disorders, parents with a personal history of an eating disorder demonstrated higher levels of Critical Comments (p <.04) (Stefanini et al., 2018). In this sample, caring for a patient with AN, rather than another type of eating disorder, was more likely to lead to increased overall caregiver burden, including the experience of anxiety and depression (p = .03). In another mixed diagnostic sample, caregivers (N = 177) of adults and adolescents with an eating disorder reported on factors posited to be associated with caregiver psychological distress, including EE, as measured by the Level of Expressed Emotion – Spanish version (LEE; Sepulveda et al., 2012, 2014). This study found increased psychological distress among carers of individuals who engaged in purging behavior compared with caregivers of patients who did not purge (p = .01). Regarding aspects of EE, for family members of patients who did not purge, a *negative attitude toward the illness*, a subscale of the LEE, was significantly associated with caregiver distress (p = .04); for families of patients who did purge, *intrusiveness* was positively associated with distress (p = .02).

The cognitive-interpersonal model of AN, first proposed in 2006 and updated in 2013 (Schmidt & Treasure, 2006; Treasure & Schmidt, 2013), highlights a pathway from caregiver distress to patient distress. In a test of this model among adolescent and adult patients with AN or EDNOS-AN (n = 152) who received inpatient or intensive outpatient treatment and their carers (n = 152), caregiver EE was significantly related to caregiver distress, which was then related to distress endorsed by patients (p <.01) (Goddard, Salerno, et al., 2013). Further, this pathway also significantly predicted eating disorder pathology (p <.01) in that patients of caregivers with greater distress experienced greater distress themselves, along with elevated scores on a measure of eating disorder behaviors and attitudes.

Using mediation analyses to further qualify associations with caregiver EE, a study of carers (N = 56), 38 of whom were caring for an adolescent or adult patient diagnosed with AN, aimed to determine predictors of caregiver burden and distress (Coomber & King, 2012). Findings indicated that caregiver EE predicted their respective experience of burden (p <.05) but not distress. Further, the association between EE and burden was fully mediated by maladaptive coping (p <.05). In another study, parents (n = 196) and adolescents receiving outpatient treatment for AN ($n = 144$) were evaluated for levels of EE, caregiver burden, and distress (Rhind et al., 2016). Results indicated that mothers demonstrated higher EOI ($p < .001$) and overall EE ($p < .01$) compared with fathers. However, mothers and fathers did not demonstrate significant differences in Critical Comments. In tests of mediation, EE did not significantly mediate the relation between time spent caregiving and distress for either mothers or fathers.

In summary, findings from the research examining characteristics of caregivers of adolescent and adult patients with AN have consistently identified elevated levels of distress and caregiver burden. Factors that may moderate or mediate these relations, such as potential differences relative to illness severity, parental psychopathology, therapeutic alliance, or parental gender, remain understudied or inconclusive, indicating a need for future inquiry.

Bidirectional Relationship in Patient and Caregiver EE

A few studies have specifically examined a patient's perspective, either by way of their interpretation of a respective caregiver's behavior, or in a dyadic view of EE. In a recent study of parents ($n = 196$) and adolescents with AN ($n = 144$), patients perceived their mothers as more overprotective and warmer than their fathers but did not discern significant differences between their two parents relative to Critical Comments (Rhind et al., 2016). Another study that tested a skills-based intervention for carers also specifically examined the perception of patients with AN regarding their caregivers' EE (Hoyle, Slater, Williams, Schmidt, & Wade, 2013). Results indicated that while there was a significant positive correlation between the caregiver and patient reports of changes in perceived EE over time ($p = .001$), ratings of the patient's perception of their parent's EE over time did not show a significant reduction.

Based on proposed models of the association between EE and relapse that conceptualize EE as a form of stress for patients, another study specifically aimed to investigate the degree to which adolescent and adult patients with transdiagnostic eating disorders ($N = 77$) may experience stress relative to their caregiver's EE (Medina-Pradas et al., 2011). Results indicated that patients perceived the attitude of their caregiver toward them as the most stressful followed by EOI. Further, patient perception of EE was related to stress and eating disorder pathology (*p*s = .04), which was not the case with caregiver perspective. Further, patient stress due to criticism related positively to eating disorder symptomatology (*p*s <.05), whereas stress associated with EOI and Warmth was not significantly associated with eating disorder symptoms.

The cognitive-interpersonal maintenance model of eating disorders identifies a core fear endorsed by patients with eating disorders in feeling criticized or judged by others (Schmidt & Treasure, 2006; Treasure & Schmidt, 2013). Further, patients with AN are more likely to endorse judging themselves by external standards, with heightened sensitivity to the reaction of others (Hambrook et al., 2011).

A recent study among families of adolescents with AN ($N = 110$) participating in an AN treatment RCT (c.f., Lock et al., 2010) created four family profiles: low patient EE/low parent EE; high patient EE/high parent EE; low patient EE/high parent EE; and high patient EE/low parent EE (Rienecke, Lebow, Lock, & Le Grange, 2017). In this study, EE was measured with the SCFI and parents were rated high in EE if they made any Critical Comments, showed any Hostility, or scored 3 or higher on EOI; patients were rated with the same criteria, with the exception of EOI. Results of this study indicated that the family EE profile was not related to remission status at end of treatment. Regarding the EE level of parents only, the low parent group (i.e., low on Critical Comments, Hostility, and EOI) demonstrated significantly lower eating pathology scores than the high parent group at the end of treatment ($p = .004$), six-month ($p = .02$), and 12-month ($p = .004$) follow-up. Overall, this study suggests that patients with AN in low-EE families do better in treatment than those patients of high-EE families, regardless of the EE status of the patient.

These study findings are notable, but to date, the investigation of patient experience of caregiver EE in AN has been considerably less than any examination of caregiver EE alone. Further, no studies have specifically examined interactions between patient and caregiver EE in impacting treatment outcome indices. Given consistent evidence that individuals with AN with primary restrictive symptoms exhibit pronounced emotion dysregulation and alexithymia (Brown et al., 2018), elevated anxiety and worry (Kaye et al., 2015), and heightened sensitivity to punishment

(Glashouwer, Bloot, Veenstra, Franken, & de Jong, 2014), further examination of patient experience of EE, as well as patient EE and its interaction with caregiver EE is a domain of needed further research.

Changes in Parental Expressed Emotion

Caregivers of individuals with AN are often distressed and may inadvertently respond to their offspring or partners in ways that contribute to the maintenance of the disorder; however, these patterns of communication may also evolve during the course of treatment. Findings from the study of changes in EE among caregivers in the context of treatment for AN have not been consistent. For example, parental criticism demonstrated increases from baseline to discharge from treatment among those receiving CFT, whereas the same domain of EE decreased among those receiving SFT (Le Grange et al., 1992). Other comparisons of CFT and SFT found that for both treatment groups, Critical Comments demonstrated a significant decrease from baseline to discharge (Eisler et al., 2000). Some work has demonstrated that both levels of criticism and EOI significantly increased over the course of treatment (Coomber & King, 2012), whereas other study findings indicated that parental EOI, but not Critical Comments, decreased after six months of treatment (Moskovich et al., 2017). Taken together, and despite discrepancies, these findings suggest that the study of how and why EE changes in the context of treatment may critically inform our understanding of treatment outcome. Interventions that are oriented toward eliciting problematic caregiver behavior in the context of eating disorder treatment are discussed more comprehensively in Chapter 7 in this volume. Accordingly, for the purposes of this chapter, this section only provides a brief summary of these findings.

Levels of EE may change naturally across the course of treatment, even when this is not the primary objective of intervention. A recent longitudinal study of adolescent patients with AN (N = 170) and their caregivers evaluated both EE and depression among caregivers (Schwarte et al., 2017). As measured by the FQ, this study qualified high EE as either a score of ≥23 on the Critical Comments scale or ≥27 on the EOI scale. Results indicated that EE and depression scores decreased over the course of treatment and that after 2.5 years, depression scores (p <.0001) and EOI (p = .0002) were still significantly lower than at admission. In contrast, Critical Comments increased significantly after discharge and at 2.5-year assessment and were comparable to levels reported at baseline. The overall finding that approximately one quarter of parents demonstrated high EE (i.e., Critical Comments) at 2.5 years following first admission suggests that EE should be evaluated during the course of treatment and beyond rather than only in the acute phase of the disorder.

Changes in EE during treatment for AN may be impacted by the age of the patient and/or independence from overall family function. A recent study aimed to investigate perceived changes in family function and caregiver EE among families of transition-age youth (TAY) patients with AN, aged 18–25, receiving family-based treatment for transition-age youth (FBT-TAY) (Dimitropoulos et al., 2018). For this study, the total score of the FQ (80) and each subscale (Critical Comments or EOI; 40) was used; a score of ≥23 on the Critical Comments scale or ≥27 on the EOI scale or a combined score of 50 was considered high. Results indicated that while family function demonstrated improvement over the course of treatment and follow-up, there were no significant changes in parental EE. Further, neither changes in perceived family functioning nor EE were associated with weight restoration or other eating disorder symptom outcomes following treatment. This study suggests that perceptions of family function may improve despite lack of change in EE. Given the unique relationship of parents and TAY, this finding is interesting and should be explored further.

Interventions Designed to Elicit Change in Expressed Emotion

Interventions designed to elicit change in EE among caregivers of those with AN have taken the form of in-person, self-help, and web-based interventions. Of in-person interventions, a study of a mixed diagnostic sample of patients with eating disorders showed an improved understanding of the eating disorder among caregivers, but this improved understanding did not seem to lessen criticism and EOI (Gísladóttir & Svavarsdóttir, 2011). Other skills-based training showed significant reductions in accommodation and enabling of some eating disorder behavior and, on the part of the caregiver, significant reduction in maladaptive coping, EE, eating disorder–specific burden, and psychological distress (Pépin & King, 2016). A more recent test of a two-session psycho-education and skills training intervention showed significant differences in decreased parent burden and Critical Comments, as well as increased parent self-efficacy, skills, and knowledge (McEvoy et al., 2019). Studies testing Experienced Carers Helping Others (ECHO), a supportive intervention that uses a book, video material, and five coaching sessions, have also demonstrated improvement in both caregiver burden and EE (Goddard et al., 2011; Hibbs et al., 2015). Notably, one of these studies also found significant improvement in patient eating pathology, quality of life, and number of days spent hospitalized as a result of this skills-based intervention (Hibbs et al., 2015).

Regarding web-based intervention, both an off-line pilot (Grover, Williams, et al., 2011), and an online RCT (Grover, Naumann, et al., 2011) of web-based cognitive-behavioral intervention for caregivers of individuals with AN or EDNOS-AN demonstrated significant reductions in caregiver anxiety, depression, and EE (measured with the LEE; Cole & Kazarian, 1993), and gains in all of these domains were maintained at follow-up (Grover, Naumann, et al., 2011). Perhaps due to sample size, one pilot feasibility study did not demonstrate changes in EE following a web-based intervention (Sepulveda et al., 2008), but preliminary findings from such interventions suggest promise and warrant further investigation. As an additional note, many of these studies have assessed change in EE in mixed diagnostic samples; given evidence that EE may differ between AN and other eating disorder diagnoses (e.g., Rienecke et al., 2016), future work may benefit from examining intervention effects on change in EE, both in person and online, uniquely for those diagnosed with AN.

Future Directions

Future work may be improved by the use of different assessment methods for EE that may provide a wider scope of understanding across its different domains. Many recent studies of EE in samples with parents of adolescents with AN have used the FQ, a validated self-report measure with the ability to assess Critical Comments and EOI (Wiedemann et al., 2002). While these domains have perhaps been the most frequently evidenced and arguably the most insidious in impacting patient experience and treatment outcomes, the FQ does not specifically assess for

Hostility, a domain that may negatively impact therapeutic alliance (Rienecke, Richmond, et al., 2016), or treatment outcome specifically in conjoint family treatment (Rienecke et al., 2016). Further, there are other aspects of interpersonal exchange encompassed within EE that deserve attention. For example, Warmth and PR, the two more positive domains of EE, may beneficially impact treatment outcomes, a possibility that has received much less research attention (Le Grange et al., 2011).

Some early work quantified high EE with pre-determined cut-offs for exhibited Hostility, Critical Comments, or EOI in the context of an interview (e.g., >1 Critical Comment; Le Grange et al., 1992), whereas other early work quantified EE with a continuous rather than a dichotomous interview score (van Furthe et al., 1996). In an effort to improve efficiency in assessment, more recent work has more often relied on self-report measures (i.e., FQ; LEE), with cut-offs pre-determined on scale scores (e.g., Dimitropoulos et al., 2018). Taken together, the extant literature in AN treatment has been reasonably consistent in implicating high(er) EE in poorer outcomes; however, systematic differences in the use of interview versus self-report or whether elevated EE is considered a category or continuous measure preclude our ability to draw comprehensive conclusions from across this research. Future work might attempt to (1) determine whether there are necessary advantages to the use of a qualitative interview format versus self-report and (2) discern more precisely whether a categorical approach to classifying EE is preferable, or alternatively, if this construct is more aptly captured as a continuous variable.

Another future direction may be to more consistently consider the role of parents individually. A substantial amount of investigation of parental EE has specifically implicated maternal EE, but some of these findings may be a result of research that has more easily recruited and studied mothers of patients with eating disorders. Work that has included both parents, with adequate statistical power to detect differences between them, has revealed unique parenting styles and needs, both of which warrant further research. Additionally, to date, no work has specifically included investigation of non-traditional households in which both parents may self-identify as the same gender or with gender fluidity.

This chapter includes a brief section on the bidirectional relationship between patient and caregiver EE. The brevity of this section underscores the dearth of research that has specifically investigated patient EE toward their parent(s), in conjunction with or interaction with caregiver EE, and its subsequent impact on treatment outcomes. While findings from a study design that includes patient EE may prove more complex and difficult to interpret, this approach may be a critical part of improving our understanding of the impact of family system dynamics on treatment outcomes.

Perhaps most critically, future research is needed to determine an improved understanding of mechanisms by which EE has an impact on AN treatment outcome. For example, future research might identify when baseline level of EE may be more important in predicting negative outcome versus when a change in EE in the context of treatment may resolve this risk; both of these options may have implications for treatment matching. Specifically, there may be particular patterns of baseline EE (e.g., high levels of Critical Comments with low Warmth) that are resistant to change in the context of family therapy, making individual or separated formats of this therapy the recommended intervention. Further, based on the medical acuity and yet chronic nature of illness among some patients with AN, identifying factors that may specifically increase Warmth and Positive Remarks and/or decrease Criticism, Hostility, or EOI over the course of treatment is a critical endeavor. Given evidence that even brief, web-based interventions may mitigate harmful aspects of EE, it remains unclear for whom and when intervention may be most indicated.

Summary and Conclusions

From its earliest published evidence over three decades ago, high EE, in particular due to Critical Comments, has demonstrated association with poorer treatment outcomes among adolescents and adults with AN. A modest but consistent line of work has suggested that in the case of high EE, a separated format of family therapy might be most helpful rather than a conjoint format of family therapy. Interventions to change EE may serve to ameliorate the increased distress and burden that are commonly evidenced among those who care for individuals with AN. Important lines of further inquiry include broader assessment of EE, inclusive of its positive domains; consideration of the unique parenting styles and needs of each parent; and improved understanding of the patients' expression *and* experience of EE. Together, answers to some of these questions may help us to understand for whom and why EE in the context of AN may lead to less promising treatment outcomes.

References

Allan, E., Le Grange, D., Sawyer, S. M., McLean, L. A., & Hughes, E. K. (2018). Parental expressed emotion during two forms of family-based treatment for adolescent anorexia nervosa. *European Eating Disorders Review*, *26*(1), 46–52.

Anastasiadou, D., Medina-Pradas, C., Sepulveda, A. R., & Treasure, J. (2014). A systematic review of family caregiving in eating disorders. *Eating Behaviors*, *15*, 464–477.

Blair, C., Freeman, C., & Cull, A. (1995). The families of anorexia nervosa and cystic fibrosis patients. *Psychological Medicine*, *25*(5), 985–993.

Blondin, S., Meilleur, D., Taddeo, D., & Frappier, J. Y. (2019). Caregiving experience and expressed emotion among parents of adolescents suffering from anorexia nervosa following illness onset. *Eating Disorders*, 1–18.

Brown, T. A., Avery, J. C., Jones, M. D., Anderson, L. K., Wierenga, C. E., & Kaye, W. H. (2018). The impact of alexithymia on emotion dysregulation in anorexia nervosa and bulimia nervosa over time. *European Eating Disorders Review*, *26*(2), 150–155.

Butzlaff, R. L., & Hooley, J. M. (1998). Expressed emotion and psychiatric relapse: A meta-analysis. *Archives of General Psychiatry*, *55*(6), 547–552.

Cole, J. D., & Kazarian, S. S. (1993). Predictive validity of the Level of Expressed Emotion (LEE) Scale: Readmission follow-up data for 1, 2, and 5-year periods. *Journal of Clinical Psychology*, *49*, 216–218.

Coomber, K., & King, R. M. (2012). Coping strategies and social support as predictors and mediators of eating disorder carer burden and psychological distress. *Social Psychiatry and Psychiatric Epidemiology*, *47*, 789–796.

Coomber, K., & King, R. M. (2013). A longitudinal examination of burden and psychological distress in carers of people with an eating disorder. *Social Psychiatry and Psychiatric Epidemiology*, *48*, 163–171.

Dimitropoulos, G., Landers, A. L., Freeman, V., Novick, J., Cullen, O., & Le Grange, D. (2018). Family-based treatment for transition age youth: The role of expressed emotion and general family functioning. *Eating Disorders*, 1–17.

Duclos, J., Dorard, G., Cook-Darzens, S., Curt, F., Faucher, S., Berthoz, S., . . . Godart, N. (2018). Predictive factors for outcome in adolescents with anorexia nervosa: To what extent does parental expressed emotion play a role? *PloS One*, *13*(7), e0196820.

Duclos, J., Vibert, S., Mattar, L., & Godart, N. (2012). Expressed emotion in families of patients with eating disorders: A review of the literature. *Current Psychiatry Reviews*, *8*(3), 183–202.

Eisler, I., Dare, C., Hodes, M., Russell, G., Dodge, E., & Le Grange, D. (2000). Family therapy for adolescent anorexia nervosa: The results of a controlled comparison of two family interventions. *The Journal of Child Psychology and Psychiatry and Allied Disciplines*, *41*(6), 727–736.

Eisler, I., Simic, M., Russell, G. F., & Dare, C. (2007). A randomised controlled treatment trial of two forms of family therapy in adolescent anorexia nervosa: A five-year follow-up. *Journal of Child Psychology and Psychiatry*, *48*(6), 552–560.

Fitzpatrick, K. K., Moye, A., Hoste, R., Lock, J., & Le Grange, D. (2010). Adolescent focused psychotherapy for adolescents with anorexia nervosa. *Journal of Contemporary Psychotherapy*, *40*(1), 31–39.

Gísladóttir, M., & Svavarsdóttir, E. K. (2011). Educational and support intervention to help families assist in the recovery of relatives with eating disorders. *Journal of Psychiatric and Mental Health Nursing*, *18*, 122–130.

Glashouwer, K. A., Bloot, L., Veenstra, E. M., Franken, I. H., & de Jong, P. J. (2014). Heightened sensitivity to punishment and reward in anorexia nervosa. *Appetite*, *75*, 97–102.

Goddard, E., Hibbs, R., Raenker, S., Salerno, L., Arcelus, J., Boughton, . . . Treasure, J. (2013). A multi-centre cohort study of short term outcomes of hospital treatment for anorexia nervosa in the UK. *BMC Psychiatry*, *13*, 287.

Goddard, E., Macdonald, P., Sepulveda, A. R., Naumann, U., Landau, S., Schmidt, U., & Treasure, J. (2011). Cognitive interpersonal maintenance model of eating disorders: Intervention for carers. *British Journal of Psychiatry*, *199*, 225–231.

Goddard, E., Salerno, L., Hibbs, R., Raenker, S., Naumann, U., Arcelus, . . . Treasure, J. (2013). Empirical examination of the interpersonal maintenance model of anorexia nervosa. *International Journal of Eating Disorders*, *46*, 867–874.

Grover, M., Naumann, U., Mohammad-Dar, L., Glennon, D., Ringwood, S., Eisler, I., . . . Schmidt, U. (2011). A randomized controlled trial of an Internet-based cognitive-behavioural skills package for carers of people with anorexia nervosa. *Psychological Medicine*, *41*, 2581–2591.

Grover, M., Williams, C., Eisler, I., Fairbairn, P., McCloskey, C., Smith, G., . . . Schmidt, U. (2011). An off-line pilot evaluation of a web-based systemic cognitive-behavioral intervention for carers of people with anorexia nervosa. *International Journal of Eating Disorders*, *44*, 708–715.

Hambrook, D., Oldershaw, A., Rimes, K., Schmidt, U., Tchanturia, K., Treasure, J., . . . Chalder, T. (2011). Emotional expression, self-silencing, and distress tolerance in anorexia nervosa and chronic fatigue syndrome. *British Journal of Clinical Psychology*, *50*(3), 310–325.

Hibbs, R., Magill, N., Goddard, E., Rhind, C., Raenker, S., Macdonald, P., . . . Treasure, J. (2015). Clinical effectiveness of a skills training intervention for caregivers in improving patient and caregiver health following in-patient treatment for severe anorexia nervosa: Pragmatic randomised controlled trial. *BJPsych Open*, *1*, 56–66.

Hoyle, D., Slater, J., Williams, C., Schmidt, U., & Wade, T. D. (2013). Evaluation of a web-based skills intervention for carers of people with anorexia nervosa: A randomized controlled trial. *International Journal of Eating Disorders*, *46*, 634–638.

Hughes, E. K., Sawyer, S. M., Accurso, E. C., Singh, S., & Le Grange, D. (2019). Predictors of early response in conjoint and separated models of family-based treatment for adolescent anorexia nervosa. *European Eating Disorders Review*, *27*(3), 283–294.

Hughes, E. K., Sawyer, S. M., Loeb, K. L., & Le Grange, D. (2015). Parent-focused treatment. In K. L. Loeb, D. Le Grange, & J. Lock (Eds.), *Family therapy for adolescent eating and weight disorders: New applications* (pp. 59–71). New York, NY: Routledge and Taylor & Francis Group.

Isserlin, L., & Couturier, J. (2012). Therapeutic alliance and family-based treatment for adolescents with anorexia nervosa. *Psychotherapy*, *49*(1), 46.

Kaye, W. H., Wierenga, C. E., Knatz, S., Liang, J., Boutelle, K., Hill, L., & Eisler, I. (2015). Temperament-based treatment for anorexia nervosa. *European Eating Disorders Review*, *23*(1), 12–18.

Kinston, W., & Loader, P. (1984). Eliciting whole-family interaction with a standardized clinical interview. *Journal of Family Therapy*, *6*, 347–363.

Leff, J. P., & Vaughn, C. E. (1985). *Expressed emotion in families: Its significance for mental illness*. New York: Guilford Press.

Le Grange, D., Eisler, I., Dare, C., & Hodes, M. (1992). Family criticism and self-starvation: A study of expressed emotion. *Journal of Family Therapy*, *14*(2), 177–192.

Le Grange, D., Eisler, I., Dare, C., & Russell, G. F. (1992). Evaluation of family treatments in adolescent anorexia nervosa: A pilot study. *International Journal of Eating Disorders, 12*(4), 347–357.

Le Grange, D., Hoste, R. R., Lock, J., & Bryson, S. W. (2011). Parental expressed emotion of adolescents with anorexia nervosa: Outcome in family-based treatment. *International Journal of Eating Disorders, 44*(8), 731–734.

Le Grange, D., Hughes, E. K., Court, A., Yeo, M., Crosby, R. D., & Sawyer, S. M. (2016). Randomized clinical trial of parent-focused treatment and family-based treatment for adolescent anorexia nervosa. *Journal of the American Academy of Child & Adolescent Psychiatry, 55*, 683–692.

Le Grange, D., Lock, J., Agras, W. S., Moye, A., Bryson, S. W., Jo, B., & Kraemer, H. C. (2012). Moderators and mediators of remission in family-based treatment and adolescent focused therapy for anorexia nervosa. *Behaviour Research and Therapy, 50*(2), 85–92.

Le Grange, D., Lock, J., Loeb, K., & Nicholls, D. (2010). Academy for eating disorders position paper: The role of the family in eating disorders. *International Journal of Eating Disorders, 43*(1), 1–5.

Lock, J., Agras, W. S., Bryson, S., & Kraemer, H. C. (2005). A comparison of short-and long-term family therapy for adolescent anorexia nervosa. *Journal of the American Academy of Child & Adolescent Psychiatry, 44*(7), 632–639.

Lock, J., & Le Grange, D. (2013). *Treatment manual for anorexia nervosa: A family-based approach*. New York: Guilford Press.

Lock, J., Le Grange, D., Agras, W. S., Moye, A., Bryson, S. W., & Jo, B. (2010). Randomized clinical trial comparing family-based treatment with adolescent-focused individual therapy for adolescents with anorexia nervosa. *Archives of General Psychiatry, 67*(10), 1025–1032.

McEvoy, P. M., Targowski, K., McGrath, D., Carter, O., Fursland, A., Fitzgerald, M., & Raykos, B. (2019). Efficacy of a brief group intervention for carers of individuals with eating disorders: A randomized control trial. *International Journal of Eating Disorders, 52*, 987–995.

Medina-Pradas, C., Navarro, J. B., Lpez, S. R., Grau, A., & Obiols, J. E. (2011). Dyadic view of expressed emotion, stress, and eating disorder psychopathology. *Appetite, 57*, 743–748.

Morgan, H. G., & Russell, G. F. M. (1975). Value of family background andclinical features as predictors of long-term outcome in anorexia nervosa: Four-year follow-up study of 41 patients. *Psychological Medicine, 5*, 355–371.

Moskovich, A. A., Timko, C. A., Honeycutt, L. K., Zucker, N. L., & Merwin, R. M. (2017). Change in expressed emotion and treatment outcome in adolescent anorexia nervosa. *Eating Disorders, 25*, 80–91.

Pépin, G., & King, R. (2016). Collaborative care skill training workshop: How Australian carers support a loved one with an eating disorder. *Advances in Eating Disorders, 4*(1), 47–58.

Rhind, C., Salerno, L., Hibbs, R., Micali, N., Schmidt, U., Gowers, S., . . . Treasure, J. (2016). The objective and subjective caregiving burden and caregiving behaviours of parents of adolescents with anorexia nervosa. *European Eating Disorders Review, 24*, 310–319.

Rienecke, R. D. (2018). Expressed emotion and eating disorders: An updated review. *Current Psychiatry Reviews, 14*(2), 84–98.

Rienecke, R. D., Accurso, E. C., Lock, J., & Le Grange, D. (2016). Expressed emotion, family functioning, and treatment outcome for adolescents with anorexia nervosa. *European Eating Disorders Review, 24*, 43–51.

Rienecke, R. D., Lebow, J., Lock, J., & Le Grange, D. (2017). Family profiles of expressed emotion in adolescent patients with anorexia nervosa and their parents. *Journal of Clinical Child & Adolescent Psychology, 46*(3), 428–436.

Rienecke, R. D., & Richmond, R. (2017). Psychopathology and expressed emotion in parents of patients with eating disorders: Relation to patient symptom severity. *Eating Disorders, 25*, 318–329.

Rienecke, R. D., Richmond, R., & Lebow, J. (2016). Therapeutic alliance, expressed emotion, and treatment outcome for anorexia nervosa in a family-based partial hospitalization program. *Eating Behaviors, 22*, 124–128.

Rienecke, R. D., Sim, L., Lock, J., & Le Grange, D. (2016). Patterns of expressed emotion in adolescent eating disorders. *Journal of Child Psychology and Psychiatry, 57*, 1407–1413.

Rutter, M., & Brown, G. W. (1966). The reliability and validity of measures of family life and relationships in families containing a psychiatric patient. *Social Psychiatry, 50*, 38–53.

Schmidt, U., & Treasure, J. (2006). Anorexia nervosa: Valued and visible: A cognitive-interpersonal maintenance model and its implications for research and practice. *British Journal of Clinical Psychology, 45*(3), 343–366.

Schwarte, R., Timmesfeld, N., Dempfle, A., Krei, M., Egberts, K., Jaite, C., . . . Bühren, K. (2017). Expressed emotions and depressive symptoms in caregivers of adolescents with first onset anorexia nervosa: A long-term investigation over 2.5 years. *European Eating Disorders Review, 25*, 44–51.

Sepulveda, A. R., Anastasiadou. D., del Maria, R. A., & Graell, M. (2012). The Spanish validation of the level of expressed emotion for relatives of people with eating disorders. *Spanish Journal of Psychology, 15*, 825–839.

Sepulveda, A. R., Anastasiadou, D., Pellegrin, Y., Andrés, P., Graell, M., Carrobles, J. A., & Morandé, G. (2014). Impact of caregiving experience on mental health among caregivers: A comparison of eating disorder patients with purging and non-purging behaviors. *Eating and Weight Disorders, 19*, 31–39.

Sepulveda, A. R., Lopez, C., Macdonald, P., & Treasure, J. (2008). Feasibility and acceptability of DVD and telephone coaching-based skills training for carers of people with an eating disorder. *International Journal of Eating Disorders, 41*, 318–325.

Stefanini, M. C., Troiani, M. R., Caselli, M., Dirindelli, P., Lucarelli, S., Caini, S., & Martinetti, M. G. (2018). Living with someone with an eating disorder: Factors affecting the caregivers' burden. *Eating and Weight Disorders-Studies on Anorexia, Bulimia and Obesity*, 1–6.

Szmukler, G. I., Eisler, I., Russell, G. F. M., & Dare, C. (1985). Anorexia nervosa, parental "expressed emotion" and dropping out of treatment. *The British Journal of Psychiatry, 147*(3), 265–271.

Treasure, J., & Schmidt, U. (2013). The cognitive-interpersonal maintenance model of anorexia nervosa revisited: A summary of the evidence for cognitive, socio-emotional and interpersonal predisposing and perpetuating factors. *Journal of Eating Disorders, 1*(1), 13.

van Furth, E. F., van Strien, D. C., Martina, L. M., van Son, M. J., Hendrickx, J. J., & van Engeland, H. (1996). Expressed emotion and the prediction of outcome in adolescent eating disorders. *International Journal of Eating Disorders, 20*(1), 19–31.

Vaughn, C. E., & Leff, J. P. (1976). The influence of family and social factors on the course of psychiatric illness: A comparison of schizophrenic and depressed neurotic patients. *The British Journal of Psychiatry, 129*(2), 125–137.

Wearden, A. J., Tarrier, N., Barrowclough, C., Zastowny, T. R., & Rahill, A. A. (2000). A review of expressed emotion research in health care. *Clinical Psychology Review, 20*(5), 633–666.

Wiedemann, G., Rayki, O., Feinstein, E., & Hahlweg, K. (2002). The family questionnaire: Development and validation of a new self-report scale for assessing expressed emotion. *Psychiatry Research, 109*(3), 265–279.

Zabala, M. J., Macdonald, P., & Treasure, J. (2009). Appraisal of caregiving burden, expressed emotion and psychological distress in families of people with eating disorders: A systematic review. *European Eating Disorders Review, 17*, 338–349.

6

EXPRESSED EMOTION AND BULIMIA NERVOSA

Renee D. Rienecke

Introduction

Although a good deal of research now exists on expressed emotion (EE) among families of individuals with anorexia nervosa (AN), perhaps less is known about EE among families of individuals with bulimia nervosa (BN). It is worth considering this diagnostic group separately, as differences have been found between families of those with AN and those with BN. A study of 181 adolescents with AN, BN, or binge eating disorder (BED) found higher levels of enmeshment and rigidity among families of patients with AN when compared with the two other groups, and families of adolescents with BN scored higher on levels of chaos and lower on levels of cohesion and flexibility than families of adolescents with AN (Cerniglia et al., 2017). A systematic review found that two studies reported no differences in eating disorder (ED) subgroups on specific elements of family functioning, while six studies found differences, including higher levels of cohesion among families of those with AN than those with BN (Holtom-Viesel & Allan, 2014).

Historically, differences in family functioning among diagnostic groups or between families with a disorder and control families were seen as playing a role in the etiology of the disorders. In the context of EDs, this is evident in Minuchin's description of the psychosomatic family

(Minuchin et al., 1975), in which families of individuals with AN and other "psychosomatic illnesses" were viewed as enmeshed, overprotective, rigid, and poor at conflict resolution. The idea that problematic family dynamics are the primary mechanisms that underlie the onset of EDs has been discredited for quite some time now (e.g., Dare, Le Grange, Eisler, & Rutherford, 1994; Le Grange, Lock, Loeb, & Nicholls, 2010), and focus has begun to shift toward viewing problematic family dynamics as a *result* of living with someone with an ED rather than the *cause* of the disorder itself (Eisler, 2005).

It is possible that families of individuals with AN and BN have different types of families. However, it is also possible that there are differences between the two diagnoses that differentially impact family functioning and family attitudes toward the illness, resulting in dissimilar levels of EE. For example, the substantial medical complications and high rates of morbidity among individuals with AN, along with the ego-syntonic nature of the disorder, could cause significant levels of stress in the family and lead to high levels of EE. For individuals with BN, the unwanted consequences of binge eating and purging behaviors (e.g., food missing that was meant for the rest of the family) could result in high levels of EE. Personality differences between patients with AN and BN could also lead to differences in EE. Although patients with EDs as a whole share certain personality traits when compared with controls, such as elevated perfectionism and neuroticism, patients with BN have been found to be more impulsive than patients with AN, exhibit more affective instability, and report more traits consistent with Cluster B personality disorders (Farstad, McGeown, & von Ranson, 2016). These associated traits could impact caregivers' views of the patient, resulting in higher levels of EE. In addition, although rates of psychiatric comorbidity are high among patients with EDs in general, rates are higher for patients with BN (94.5%) than AN (56.2%) (Hudson, Hiripi, Pope, & Kessler, 2007), possibly resulting in higher levels of caregiver EE among relatives of patients with BN.

EE is a long-term predictor of caregiver burden (Coomber & King, 2013, see also Chapter 7, this volume), which has been found to be substantial among carers of individuals with AN, with carers reporting higher levels of difficulties than carers of individuals with psychosis

(Treasure et al., 2001) and high levels of unmet needs, including needing information about EDs, needing support from other people or organizations, and needing information from general practitioners (Haigh & Treasure, 2003). Less is known about the caregiving experiences of carers of individuals with BN. A qualitative study of 20 caregivers found several themes emerging from the interviews, including the process of detection of the illness and the impact this had on caregivers, such as feelings of helplessness and feeling that they should have identified the problem sooner (Perkins, Winn, Murray, Murphy, & Schmidt, 2004). Additional themes included a range of emotional and physical responses, such as self-blame and exhaustion, practical difficulties such as managing meals and affording groceries, concern about the relationship with the individual with BN, and finding coping strategies. Positive aspects of the caregiving experience included feeling that the illness had brought the caregiver and patient closer together. Similar to carers of individuals with AN, carers of individuals with BN reported needing more information on EDs and treatment, better access to treatment, and an outlet to talk about their difficulties (Winn, Perkins, Murray, Murphy, & Schmidt, 2004).

In a direct comparison of caregivers of AN versus BN, Graap et al. (2008) found that carers of individuals with BN reported fewer problems and needs compared with carers of individuals with AN or schizophrenia, and another study found that subjective burden was lower among caregivers of those with BN than AN (Santonastaso, Saccon, & Favaro, 1997). Caring for an individual with AN is also associated with higher scores on a measure of accommodating and enabling behaviors when compared with carers of individuals with BN (Stefanini et al., 2018). Although the number of patients with BN was small in these studies, it is possible that caregiver burden is lower among carers of individuals with BN. However, the presence of purging behaviors among patients has been found to be one of the most important predictors of low caregiver quality of life (Martín et al., 2011), and distress is higher among caregivers of patients with purging behaviors than caregivers of patients with non-purging behaviors (Sepulveda et al., 2014). Thus, the evidence for caregiver burden is somewhat mixed. Negative aspects of caregiving are associated with high EE among carers of individuals with AN (Kyriacou, Treasure, & Schmidt, 2008). It will be informative to examine EE separately among carers of individuals with BN to better understand possible differences in family attitudes toward illness and illness-related behaviors across diagnoses. The following sections outline what is known about EE in the context of BN, contrasting with other disorders when possible.

Expressed Emotion and BN

Several studies have examined EE among caregivers of individuals with EDs, but many examine caregiver characteristics as a whole rather than comparing across diagnostic subgroups. One of the earliest studies to compare parents of patients with AN or BN examined EE using the Camberwell Family Interview (CFI) with 40 mothers and 35 fathers of 51 patients with AN or BN (Szmukler, Eisler, Russell, & Dare, 1985). Both mothers and fathers were more critical of patients with BN, and fathers of patients with BN scored higher on Emotional Overinvolvement (EOI) than fathers of patients with AN. A small study comparing a group of 18 patients with AN to eight patients with BN, also using the Camberwell Family Interview (CFI), found that mothers of patients with BN scored higher on Warmth and on Critical Comments, but neither of these findings was statistically significant (Dare et al., 1994). Another small study compared nine patients with AN, 12 patients with BN, and three patients with ED not otherwise specified (EDNOS). EE was examined with the Family Problems Questionnaire (Morosini et al., 1991), which has two EE subscales: hypercriticism and overinvolvement. The authors found that relatives of patients with AN rated themselves higher on overinvolvement than relatives of patients with BN. Criticism was also higher among relatives of patients with AN, but the difference between the groups was not significant (Santonastaso et al., 1997). A study of 97 carers of 62 patients with AN and ten with BN also found no differences in EE scores between the two groups (Stefanini et al., 2018). Another study using the CFI did not report differences in parental EE between patients with BN and those with AN but found that fathers had higher rates of hostility toward patients who were using laxatives than those who were not (van Furth et al., 1996).

A larger study examined EE among 197 carers of patients with AN, 82 carers of patients with BN, and 43 carers of patients with major depressive disorder (MDD) (Rienecke, Sim, Lock, & Le Grange, 2016). EE was assessed with the Standardized Clinical Family Interview (SCFI) (Kinston & Loader, 1984). The SCFI can be used to assess the five original subscales of EE and is comparable to the CFI (Brown & Rutter, 1966; Hodes, Dare, Dodge, & Eisler, 1999; Vaughn & Leff, 1976), which is the gold-standard assessment tool for rating EE, but is shorter to administer and score. Fathers were found to make more Critical Comments toward patients with BN or MDD than toward patients with AN. Family status was also investigated in this study, and fathers from non-intact families made more Critical Comments toward patients with BN than fathers from intact families. Mothers also made more Critical Comments toward patients with BN than AN and made more Critical Comments toward patients with BN than MDD. Mothers made more positive remarks toward patients with AN or BN than MDD.

In one of the few longitudinal investigations of EE, 30 inpatients with BN who were either low or high on EE were followed over the course of six years (Hedlund, Fichter, Quadflieg, & Brandl, 2003). Patients were assessed at four time points: at admission to the inpatient unit, upon discharge from the hospital, at two-year follow-up, and at six-year follow-up. The CFI was conducted at admission and used to classify patients as high or low on EE based on their caregivers' scores on the subscales of Critical Comments and EOI. The Family Environment Scale (FES) (Moos & Moos, 1986) consists of ten subscales assessing various aspects of family environment, and the Beck Depression Inventory (BDI) (Beck, Ward, Mendelson, Mock, & Erbaugh, 1961) was used to measure depression. The Structured Interview for Anorexia and Bulimia Nervosa (SIAB) (Fichter et al., 1991) was used at both follow-up assessments, and the Eating Disorder Inventory (EDI) (Garner, Olmsted, & Polivy, 1983) was administered at all four time points.

No differences were found for mood, anxiety, or personality disorders between patients from low versus high-EE families, and there was no difference in body mass index (BMI) between low- and high-EE patients at any time point. Scores on the SIAB and EDI showed that patients from high-EE families had consistently and significantly more eating-disordered behaviors and cognitions than patients from low-EE families, as well as higher levels of depression. Patients from high-EE families also reported more conflict and less organization in their families. This suggests the utility of family EE status as an outcome predictor, even six years later.

Another longitudinal investigation assessed EE at baseline (T1), 4.5 months (T2), and nine months (T3) among 56 carers of patients with EDs, seven of whom had BN (Coomber & King, 2013). Critical Comments as measured by the Family Questionnaire (FQ) (Wiedemann, Rayki, Feinstein, & Hahlweg, 2002) did not change from T1 to T3, but EOI decreased. EE was a significant predictor of carer burden from T1 to T2, and the relationship between EE and burden has been found to be mediated by maladaptive coping (Coomber & King, 2012). Findings suggest that parental criticism may be fairly stable over time, which has been found in other populations (Peris & Baker, 2000), although one study found that EE was stable among fathers but not among mothers, whose EE level was more influenced by stressful situations (Santos et al., 2001).

Several studies have examined perceived EE, suggesting that the perception of the ill relative is also important to the understanding of EE, in addition to objective or self-report ratings. A study assessing perceived EE using the Level of Expressed Emotion (LEE) Scale among 20 patients with AN, 20 with BN, and 23 with BED found no differences across diagnostic subgroups (DiPaola, Faravelli, & Ricca, 2010). Another study examined patients' levels of stress due to carers' EE (using the Perceived Stress due to Expressed Emotion scale), patients' perceived EE (using the Brief Dyadic Scale of Expressed Emotion), and objectively rated EE (using the CFI) and found no differences between patients with AN and BN (Medina-Pradas, Navarro, López, Grau, & Obiols, 2011). EE as rated by the patient has been found to predict a negative experience of caregiving among carers of patients with BN (Winn et al., 2007).

Patients' perception of EE is important to take into consideration, as it may impact choice of treatment or treatment format. In a study of 85 adolescent patients with BN or EDNOS-BN who were randomized to either family therapy or cognitive-behavioral guided self-care, patients were required to choose a close other to participate in either treatment (Perkins et al., 2005). A sizable minority (27%) of patients chose not to include either parent in their treatment. In addition to being older, having a longer duration of illness, and having higher rates of depression and more comorbid and impulsive behaviors, those who chose not to include their parents in treatment rated their mothers as higher on EE on the LEE Scale than patients who chose to include their parents.

Family EE Profiles and BN

The majority of work in EE has rated relatives' attitudes and behaviors toward an ill family member or has rated the ill family member's perception of his or her relatives' EE level. One study has examined the overall family profile of patients with BN and their caregivers by rating EE from patients toward parents.

In a treatment study of 54 adolescents with BN and their families, the SCFI was administered at baseline. EE ratings were made from parents to patients but were also made from patients to parents, with the exception of the EOI scale. Patients and parents were classified as high or low on EE, and families were then placed into four family EE profiles: high patient/high parent, high patient/low parent, low patient/high parent, and low patient/low parent (Hoste, Lebow, & Le Grange, 2015).

Outcome was assessed by examining percent reduction in binge eating and purging after one year of treatment. While there were no significant differences between groups in reduction of binge eating behaviors, the Low Patient/Low Parent group showed the greatest reduction in purging (81.9%) at the end of treatment. Given what is known about the impact of high EE on treatment outcome in the EDs, this was perhaps not a surprising finding. Interestingly, however, the group with the next-highest reduction in purging was the High Patient/High Parent group (73.7%). This prompted the authors to combine patients and parents into matched (Low Patient/Low Parent plus High Patient/High Parent) and unmatched (Low Patient/High Parent plus High Patient/Low Parent) groups and found that the matched groups had a significantly higher reduction in purging (80.1%) than the unmatched groups (54.7%).

It is intriguing to consider whether the match in EE level between patient and parent may be important for individuals with BN, particularly as a similar study found that this was not the case among families of patients with AN (Rienecke, Lebow, Lock, & Le Grange, 2017). The authors suggest that personality differences sometimes found among patients with AN versus BN (c.f., Kaye, Fudge, & Paulus, 2009; Steiger & Bruce, 2004; Wonderlich, Lilenfeld, Riso, Engel, & Mitchell, 2005) may enable patients with BN to weather higher levels of parental emotions such as criticism, whereas patients with AN may be more sensitive to parental criticism, thus faring better with parents who are low on EE. This is consistent with findings that family hassles (e.g., restrictions at home such as early curfew) predicted bulimic episodes for patients who perceived their family to be low on emotional expressiveness, but this was not true for patients who perceived their families to be high on emotional expressiveness (Okon, Greene, & Smith, 2003).

Interventions for Caregivers of Patients With BN

A four-week educational and support intervention was offered to 24 caregivers of 14 patients, the majority of whom (57%) had BN (Gísladóttir & Svavarsdóttir, 2011). The intervention was based on the Calgary Family Intervention Model (CFIM) (Wright & Leahey, 2009) and involved educational lectures; tasks to be completed in session and between sessions, such as active listening; and support intervention and conversation, such as assessing the impact of the illness on the family. EE was measured with the LEE scale, a self-report questionnaire that assesses four subscales – intrusiveness, emotional response, attitude toward illness/understanding, and tolerance/expectations (Cole & Kazarian, 1988) – and the FQ. The authors found a significant improvement in the "understanding" subscale of the LEE from pre- to post-treatment. Several other subscales on the LEE and FQ improved, but changes were not statistically significant. Caregivers also reported an improvement on the subscale of "eating behavior, concern with weight and food, denial of problem" on the Anorectic Behavior Observation Scale (ABOS) (Vandereycken, 1992). However, it is unclear if this improvement in eating disordered behavior was due to a decrease in caregiver EE, as the patients were in treatment at the time.

A psychoeducational intervention for 28 relatives of 26 patients, seven of whom had BN, found that rates of high EE relatives decreased significantly after five two-hour sessions focused on psychoeducation and group discussion (Uehara, Kawashima, Goto, Tasaki, & Someya, 2001). However, Critical Comments and patients' symptoms did not change. Comparisons between diagnostic groups were not made in this study. Additional studies of interventions have included carers of patients with

BN but have not reported outcomes separately for diagnostic subgroups (e.g., Goddard et al., 2011; Pépin & King, 2013; Sepulveda et al., 2010).

Ethnic Differences in EE

One study has examined ethnic differences in EE among families of patients with BN (Hoste & Le Grange, 2008). Eighty-four carers of 55 adolescent patients with BN participated in the SCFI. Patients identifying as white were compared with patients identifying as members of an ethnic minority group. Half of patients in the minority group were classified as high on EE compared with 28% of patients in the white group, but this difference was not statistically significant, and no other differences were found between the groups of families.

Conclusions and Future Directions

The majority of work on caregivers of patients with EDs has been on adolescents and adults with AN, with only a few studies examining caregivers of patients with BN. Several studies have found few differences in EE between caregivers of patients with AN and BN, although larger studies have found that both mothers and fathers are more critical toward patients with BN than AN. Perceived EE, measured by the patient, does not seem to differ between diagnostic groups. EE does seem to be a useful predictor of treatment outcome over time, as well as caregiver burden.

Hodes and Le Grange (1993) have suggested several possible reasons for higher levels of criticism among parents of patients with BN as compared wth those with AN. Parents of patients with AN may in some ways approve of their child's degree of restriction, particularly if that parent has dieted in the past. The rigidity and orderliness of AN may provoke less criticism from parents than the unpredictability or apparent willful nature of BN behavior, and the clear frailty of a patient with AN may lead parents to be more protective than critical. Binge eating and purging behaviors may also be seen as more disruptive to family life than restricting behaviors. Further research on parents' perceptions of their child's illness would be helpful to better understand the reasons behind parental criticism, particularly as parental attributions about illness-related behaviors have been shown to be associated with EE in the context of schizophrenia (Barrowclough, Johnston, & Tarrier, 1994; Brewin, MacCarthy,

Duda, & Vaughn, 1991; Leff & Vaughn, 1985). High-EE relatives attribute unwanted behaviors to the patient, rather than the illness, while low-EE relatives see the illness as genuine and are more empathic toward the patient. It is possible that caregivers of patients with BN view the illness differently than caregivers of patients with AN.

There is also a need for further studies on the effectiveness of interventions designed to reduce EE among caregivers of those with BN, as well as further research on the match between patient and parent EE, how it is related to treatment outcome, and whether the pattern differs depending on diagnosis. Future research may also benefit from an examination of specific ways in which EE contributes to poor treatment outcome. In one study of dieting concerns and binge eating in college women, the authors found that perceived parental criticism was associated with external attributions of control and depression, which in turn were associated with increased disordered eating behaviors (Meno, Hannum, Espelage, & Low, 2008), and Sassaroli et al. (2011) found that perfectionism had a mediating effect on the relationship between perceived parental criticism and drive for thinness. Peris and Miklowitz (2015) suggest that EE is a form of "toxic family stress" – a problematic response to psychiatric illness that may exacerbate symptoms. The authors suggest that emotionally charged family interactions may worsen the illness and make recovery more difficult over time, thus perpetuating parental criticism and EOI while parents struggle to effectively respond to and care for their child. A better understanding of the mechanisms by which high EE leads to poor outcome for EDs may inform efforts to develop effective interventions.

References

Barrowclough, C., Johnston, M., & Tarrier, N. (1994). Attributions, expressed emotion, and patient relapse: An attributional model of relatives' response to schizophrenic illness. *Behavior Therapy*, *25*, 67–88.

Beck, A. T., Ward, C. H., Mendelson, M., Mock, J., & Erbaugh, J. (1961). An inventory for measuring depression. *Archives of General Psychiatry*, *4*, 561–571.

Brewin, C. R., MacCarthy, B., Duda, K., & Vaughn, C. E. (1991). Attribution and expressed emotion in the relatives of patients with schizophrenia. *Journal of Abnormal Psychology*, *100*, 546–554.

Brown, G. W., & Rutter, M. (1966). The measurement of family activities and relationships: A methodological study. *Human Relations*, *19*, 241–263.

Cerniglia, L., Cimino, S., Tafà, M., Marzilli, E., Ballarotto, G., & Bracaglia, F. (2017). Family profiles in eating disorders: Family functioning and psychopathology. *Psychology Research and Behavior Management*, *10*, 305–312.

Cole, J. D., & Kazarian, S. S. (1988). The level of expressed emotion scale: A new measure of expressed emotion. *Journal of Clinical Psychology, 44*, 392–397.
Coomber, K., & King, R. M. (2012). Coping strategies and social support as predictors and mediators of eating disorder carer burden and psychological distress. *Social Psychiatry & Psychiatric Epidemiology, 47*, 789–796.
Coomber, K., & King, R. M. (2013). A longitudinal examination of burden and psychological distress in carers of people with an eating disorder. *Social Psychiatry & Psychiatric Epidemiology, 48*, 163–171.
Dare, C., Le Grange, D., Eisler, I., & Rutherford, J. (1994). Redefining the psychosomatic family: Family process of 26 eating disorder families. *International Journal of Eating Disorders, 16*, 211–226.
DiPaola, F., Faravelli, C., & Ricca, V. (2010). Perceived expressed emotion in anorexia nervosa, bulimia nervosa, and binge-eating disorder. *Comprehensive Psychiatry, 51*, 401–405.
Eisler, I. (2005). The empirical and theoretical base of family therapy and multiple family day therapy for adolescent anorexia nervosa. *Journal of Family Therapy, 27*, 104–131.
Farstad, S. M., McGeown, L. M., & von Ranson, K. M. (2016). Eating disorders and personality, 2004–2016: A systematic review and meta-analysis. *Clinical Psychology Review, 46*, 91–105.
Fichter, M. M., Elton, M., Engel, K., Meyer, A. E., Mall, H., & Poustka, F. (1991). Structured Interview for Anorexia and Bulimia Nervosa (SIAB): Development of a new instrument for the assessment of eating disorders. *International Journal of Eating Disorders, 10*, 571–592.
Garner, D. M., Olmsted, M. P., & Polivy, J. (1983). Development and validation of a multidimensional Eating Disorder Inventory for anorexia nervosa and bulimia. *International Journal of Eating Disorders, 2*, 15–34.
Gísladóttir, M., & Svavarsdóttir, E. K. (2011). Educational and support intervention to help families assist in the recovery of relatives with eating disorders. *Journal of Psychiatric and Mental Health Nursing, 18*, 122–130.
Goddard, E., Macdonald, P., Sepulveda, A. R., Naumann, U., Landau, S., Schmidt, U., & Treasure, J. (2011). Cognitive interpersonal maintenance model of eating disorders: Intervention for carers. *The British Journal of Psychiatry, 199*, 225–231.
Graap, H., Bleich, S., Herbst, F., Scherzinger, C., Trostmann, Y., Wancata, J., & de Zwaan, M. (2008). The needs of carers: A comparison between eating disorders and schizophrenia. *Social Psychiatry and Psychiatric Epidemiology, 43*, 800–807.
Haigh, R., & Treasure, J. (2003). Investigating the needs of carers in the area of eating disorders: Development of the Carers' Needs Assessment Measure (CaNAM). *European Eating Disorders Review, 11*, 125–141.
Hedlund, S., Fichter, M. M., Quadflieg, N., & Brandl, C. (2003). Expressed emotion, family environment, and parental bonding in bulimia nervosa: A 6-year investigation. *Eating and Weight Disorders, 8*, 26–35.
Hodes, M., Dare, C., Dodge, E., & Eisler, I. (1999). The assessment of expressed emotion in a standardized family interview. *Journal of Child Psychology and Psychiatry, 40*, 617–625.
Hodes, M., & Le Grange, D. (1993). Expressed emotion in the investigation of eating disorders: A review. *International Journal of Eating Disorders, 13*, 279–288.
Holtom-Viesel, A., & Allan, S. (2014). A systematic review of the literature on family functioning across all eating disorder diagnoses in comparison to control families. *Clinical Psychology Review, 34*, 29–43.
Hoste, R. R., Lebow, J., & Le Grange, D. (2015). A bidirectional examination of expressed emotion among families of adolescents with bulimia nervosa. *International Journal of Eating Disorders, 48*, 249–252.

Hoste, R. R., & Le Grange, D. (2008). Expressed emotion among white and ethnic minority families of adolescents with bulimia nervosa. *European Eating Disorders Review, 16*, 395–400.
Hudson, J. I., Hiripi, E., Pope, H. G., Jr., & Kessler, R. C. (2007). The prevalence and correlates of eating disorders in the National Comorbidity Survey Replication. *Biological Psychiatry, 61*, 348–358.
Kaye, W. H., Fudge, J. L., & Paulus, M. (2009). New insights into symptoms and neurocircuit function of anorexia nervosa. *Nature Reviews Neuroscience, 10*, 573–584.
Kinston, W., & Loader, P. (1984). Eliciting whole-family interaction with a standardized clinical interview. *Journal of Family Therapy, 6*, 347–363.
Kyriacou, O., Treasure, J., & Schmidt, U. (2008). Expressed emotion in eating disorders assessed via self-report: An examination of factors associated with expressed emotion in carers of people with anorexia nervosa in comparison to control families. *International Journal of Eating Disorders, 41*, 37–46.
Leff, J., & Vaughn, C. (1985). *Expressed emotion in families: Its significance for mental illness.* New York: Guilford Press.
Le Grange, D., Lock, J., Loeb, K., & Nicholls, D. (2010). Academy for eating disorders position paper: The role of the family in eating disorders. *International Journal of Eating Disorders, 43*, 1–5.
Martín, J., Padierna, A., Aguirre, U., Quintana, J. M., Las Hayas, C., & Muñoz, P. (2011). Quality of life among caregivers of patients with eating disorders. *Quality of Life Research, 20*, 1359–1369.
Medina-Pradas, C., Navarro, J. B., López, S. R., Grau, A., & Obiols, J. E. (2011). Dyadic view of expressed emotion, stress, and eating disorder psychopathology. *Appetite, 57*, 743–748.
Meno, C. A., Hannum, J. W., Espelage, D. E., & Low, K. S. D. (2008). Familial and individual variables as predictors of dieting concerns and binge eating in college females. *Eating Behaviors, 9*, 91–101.
Minuchin, S., Baker, L., Rosman, B. L., Liebman, R., Milman, L., & Todd, T. C. (1975). A conceptual model of psychosomatic illness in children: Family organization and family therapy. *Archives of General Psychiatry, 32*, 1031–1038.
Moos, R. H., & Moos, B. S. (1986). *Family environment scale manual* (2nd ed.). Palo Alto: Consulting Psychologists Press.
Morosini, P., Roncone, R., Veltro, F., Palomba, U., & Casacchia, M. (1991). Routine assessment tool in psychiatry: A case of questionnaire of family attitudes and burden. *Italian Journal of Psychiatry and Behavioural Sciences, 1*, 95–101.
Okon, D. M., Greene, A. L., & Smith, J. E. (2003). Family interactions predict intraindividual symptom variation for adolescents with bulimia. *International Journal of Eating Disorders, 34*, 450–457.
Pépin, G., & King, R. (2013). Collaborative care skills training workshops: Helping carers cope with eating disorders from the UK to Australia. *Social Psychiatry and Psychiatric Epidemiology, 48*, 805–812.
Peris, T. S., & Baker, B. L. (2000). Applications of the expressed emotion construct to young children with externalizing behavior: Stability and prediction over time. *Journal of Child Psychology and Psychiatry, 41*, 457–462.
Peris, T. S., & Miklowitz, D. J. (2015). Parental expressed emotion and youth psychopathology: New directions for an old construct. *Child Psychiatry & Human Development, 46*, 863–873.
Perkins, S., Schmidt, U., Eisler, I., Treasure, J., Yi, I., Winn, S., . . . Berelowitz, M. (2005). Why do adolescents with bulimia nervosa choose not to involve their parents in treatment? *European Child & Adolescent Psychiatry, 14*, 376–385.

Perkins, S., Winn, S., Murray, J., Murphy, R., & Schmidt, U. (2004). A qualitative study of the experience of caring for a person with bulimia nervosa, Part 1: The emotional impact of caring. *International Journal of Eating Disorders, 36*, 256–268.
Rienecke, R. D., Lebow, J., Lock, J., & Le Grange, D. (2017). Family profiles of expressed emotion in adolescent patients with anorexia nervosa and their parents. *Journal of Clinical Child & Adolescent Psychology, 46*, 428–436.
Rienecke, R. D., Sim, L., Lock, J., & Le Grange, D. (2016). Patterns of expressed emotion in adolescent eating disorders. *Journal of Child Psychology and Psychiatry, 57*, 1407–1413.
Santonastaso, P., Saccon, D., & Favaro, A. (1997). Burden and psychiatric symptoms on key relatives of patients with eating disorders: A preliminary study. *Eating and Weight Disorders, 1*, 44–48.
Santos, A., Espina, A., Pumar, B., González, P., Ayerbe, A., & García, E. (2001). Longitudinal study of the stability of expressed emotion in families of schizophrenic patients: A 9-month follow-up. *The Spanish Journal of Psychology, 4*, 65–71.
Sassaroli, S., Apparigliato, M., Bertelli, S., Boccalari, L., Fiore, F., Lamela, C., . . . Ruggiero, G. M. (2011). Perfectionism as a mediator between perceived criticism and eating disorders. *Eating and Weight Disorders, 16*, e37–e44.
Sepulveda, A. R., Anastasiadou, D., Pellegrin, Y., Andrés, P., Graell, M., Carrobles, J. A., & Morandé, G. (2014). Impact of caregiving experience on mental health among caregivers: A comparison of eating disorder patients with purging and non-purging behaviors. *Eating and Weight Disorders, 19*, 31–39.
Sepulveda, A. R., Todd, G., Whitaker, W., Grover, M., Stahl, D., & Treasure, J. (2010). Expressed emotion in relatives of patients with eating disorders following skills training program. *International Journal of Eating Disorders, 43*, 603–610.
Stefanini, M. C., Troiani, M. R., Caselli, M., Dirindelli, P., Lucarelli, S., Caini, S., & Martinetti, M. G. (2018). Living with someone with an eating disorder: Factors affecting the caregivers' burden. *Eating and Weight Disorders*. doi:10.1007/s40519-018-0480-7
Steiger, H., & Bruce, K. Personality traits and disorders in anorexia nervosa, bulimia nervosa and binge eating disorder. In T. D. Brewerton (Ed.), *Clinical handbook of eating disorders: An integrated approach* (pp. 207–228). New York, NY: Marcel Dekker Inc.
Szmukler, G. I., Eisler, I., Russell, G. F. M., & Dare, C. (1985). Anorexia nervosa, parental "expressed emotion" and dropping out of treatment. *British Journal of Psychiatry, 147*, 265–271.
Treasure, J., Murphy, T., Szmukler, G., Todd, G., Gavan, K., & Joyce, J. (2001). The experience of caregiving for severe mental illness: A comparison between anorexia nervosa and psychosis. *Social Psychiatry and Psychiatric Epidemiology, 36*, 343–347.
Uehara, T., Kawashima, Y., Goto, M., Tasaki, S., & Someya, T. (2001). Psychoeducation for the families of patients with eating disorders and changes in expressed emotion: A preliminary study. *Comprehensive Psychiatry, 42*, 132–138.
Vandereycken, W. (1992). Validity and reliability of the anorectic behavior observation scale for parents. *Acta Psychiatrica Scandinavica, 85*, 163–166.
van Furth, E. F., van Strien, D. C., Martina, L. M. L., van Son, M. J. M., Hendrickx, J. J. P., & van Engeland, H. (1996). Expressed emotion and the prediction of outcome in adolescent eating disorders. *International Journal of Eating Disorders, 20*, 19–31.
Vaughn, C. E., & Leff, J. P. (1976). The measurement of expressed emotion in the families of psychiatric patients. *British Journal of Social and Clinical Psychology, 15*, 157–165.
Wiedemann, G., Rayki, O., Feinstein, E., & Hahlweg, K. (2002). The family questionnaire: Development and validation of a new self-report scale for assessing expressed emotion. *Psychiatry Research, 109*, 265–279.

Winn, S., Perkins, S., Murray, J., Murphy, R., & Schmidt, U. (2004). A qualitative study of the experience of caring for a person with bulimia nervosa, Part 2: Carers' needs and experiences of services and other support. *International Journal of Eating Disorders, 36*, 269–279.
Winn, S., Perkins, S., Walwyn, R., Schdmit, U., Eisler, I., Treasure, J., . . . Yi, I. (2007). Predictors of mental health problems and negative caregiving experiences in carers of adolescents with bulimia nervosa. *International Journal of Eating Disorders, 40*, 171–178.
Wonderlich, S. A., Lilenfeld, L. R., Riso, L. P., Engel, S., & Mitchell, J. E. (2005). Personality and anorexia nervosa. *International Journal of Eating Disorders, 37*, S68–S71.
Wright, M., & Leahey, M. (2009). The calgary family intervention model. In M. Wright & M. Leahey (Eds.), *Nurses and families: A guide to family assessment and intervention* (5th ed., pp. 153–179). Philadelphia, PA: F. A. Davis Company.

7

Emotionally Driven Behaviors (Expressed Emotion, Accommodating, Enabling, and Splitting) and How to Manage Them in the Social Network of People With Eating Disorders

Janet Treasure, Dan Willmott, and Valentina Cardi

Introduction

The widespread experience or perception of solitude is deeply connected to the development and maintenance of anorexia nervosa. This is epitomized in a poignant and revealing quote from the personal journey of a doctor with lived experience of the illness: "I was recently asked to sum up my experience of anorexia nervosa in one sentence – actually, I can do it in just one word – **isolation**" (McKnight & Boughton, 2014). It emphasizes how loneliness (Levine, 2012) and problems in social and vocational functioning are outcomes from the illness, which are of key relevance for patients themselves (Harrison, Mountford, & Tchanturia, 2014). Family-based treatment (FBT) (recommended by most guidelines as a first-line treatment for adolescents) overcomes this tendency towards social alienation by drawing in family members to provide support. In contrast, treatments for adults with anorexia nervosa have not placed such an emphasis on building social resources and social support. Indeed, carers often complain that they are excluded from treatment (Haigh & Treasure, 2003).

In the seminal study of FBT, Russell stratified participants into subgroups based on age and the duration of their illness (Russell, Szmukler, Dare, & Eisler, 1987). Interestingly, FBT reduced relapse following inpatient care only in young adolescents with a short illness duration. It is perhaps easy to understand why an approach, in which parents take total control of meals, is less of a good fit for the management of adults with anorexia nervosa. Indeed, when FBT was modified for adults, the outcomes were comparable to specialist, individual therapies (Eisler et al., 1997). However, the intriguing question as to why adolescents with a protracted illness are resistant to FBT needs to be considered. The original premise of FBT was that it was agnostic as to aetiology. However, best practice in modern medicine is to use individualized treatment to target aetiological and/or maintaining factors. Developments in neuroscience and psychosocial research have produced insight into the factors that predispose to an eating disorder and more important, given the protracted clinical course, factors that maintain the illness. One possible answer to the 'why' questions of treatment resistance is that interpersonal maintaining factors develop during the evolution of the illness and lead to social alienation.

The Cognitive Interpersonal Model

The cognitive interpersonal model was developed from clinical and neuroscience evidence (Schmidt & Treasure, 2006; Treasure & Schmidt, 2013). The model posits that anomalies in social cognition are a mechanism underpinning the interpersonal problems recognized as predisposing and perpetuating factors in anorexia nervosa (Caglar-Nazali et al., 2014). The initial description of the model emphasized the valuable and visible aspects of the disorder. The later iteration of the model details more of the supporting neuroscience (Treasure & Schmidt, 2013). A summary of the interpersonal component of the model is shown in Figure 7.1.

The Emotional Reactions of Close Others (the Visible Impact of Anorexia Nervosa)

The highly visible and socially disruptive signs and symptoms of anorexia nervosa produce a profound impact on others (see Figure 7.1 and Table 7.1).

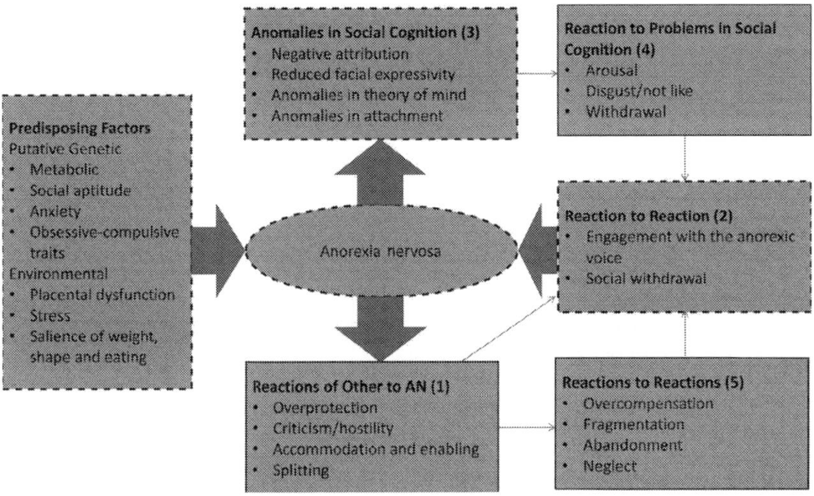

Figure 7.1 The interpersonal element of the cognitive interpersonal model. The dashed lines represent the person with anorexia nervosa, and the solid lines represent close others. The dashed/dotted lines represent predisposing factors, whereas the other boxes represent factors that build from the illness and act to maintain the illness.

Table 7.1 The reaction of close others to ED behaviors

Why	What	Who and When
Anxiety because of overt signs or symptoms of starvation	Overprotection; allowances because of the sick role	Carer in early stage
Frustration at refusal to adopt the obvious simple solution (i.e. to eat) Anger at antisocial behaviors (withdrawal from social eating, lying, cheating, etc)	Hostility and criticism	Carer in early stage
Reduced efficacy and high anxiety: adaptation and acceptance of status quo	Accommodating behavior; joining in or allowing with eating disorder rules	Carer in late stage
Adjustment or acceptance and concern about social impact	Enabling behavior (e.g. providing money for food, covering up for negative consequences)	Carer in late stage
Counter reactions in co-parent (e.g. overprotection, withdrawal, hostility) Counter reactions of sibling or partner (e.g. anger, stress, abandonment)	Interpersonal tension, opposition, withdrawal, or fragmentation	Dyads within the family
Shame, stigma, or accommodation	Secrecy and family isolation	Family as a unit

Sharing food is one of the cornerstones of social behavior, and mealtimes are significant for cultural and symbolic reasons; therefore, withdrawal from this custom is highly disruptive. Furthermore, some of the strategies undertaken in pursuit of eating disorder goals are fundamentally antisocial; in following the anorexic voice and pursuing eating disorder rules, people with anorexia nervosa can resort to arguing, lying, cheating, and stealing and do not register the antisocial impact this has on close others. They may be unaware that the signals they are sending include expressions of disgust towards food and those that provide it. It is not surprising that these behaviors elicit Critical Comments, Hostility and a lack of Warmth from others, especially as the solution to the problems that anorexia has caused is simple: "just eat". In addition, the skeletal form and obvious signs of illness evoke horror and anxiety in close others. This elicits a powerful caregiving response; an overprotective reaction to the sick role, leading to accommodating behavior in the anxious caregivers.

Accommodation refers to changes that families or close others make to their own behavior with the intention of helping someone with a mental health disorder assuage distress related to their illness. In the short term, this is effective as it can temporarily reduce anxiety (for example, through excessive reassurance or by giving into eating disorder demands) but over time places tremendous burden on caregivers, negatively impacts their quality of life, and is associated with more entrenched eating disorder symptomatology (Anastasiadou, Medina-Pradas, Sepulveda, & Treasure, 2014; Lebowitz, Panza, & Bloch, 2016). These patterns of interactions become ingrained as they are negatively reinforcing for the patient (by directly reducing distress) and the caregiver (by reducing distress related to seeing the patient's own emotional distress).

It is common for an individual to oscillate between these two styles of emotional responses (namely, hostility and accommodation). Alternatively, one caregiver will fall into one style, and the other may counter any extreme response by going to the opposite emotional pole. The diversity of these reactions fragments the caregiving response to the illness, allowing eating disorder behaviors to flourish. Certainly, high expressed emotion is common in parents of eating disorder sufferers, with 64% showing high Emotional Overinvolvement (EOI) and 47% showing high criticism (compared with 3% and 15%, respectively, in parents of healthy controls) (Kyriacou, Treasure, & Schmidt, 2008; Whitney et al., 2005).

Reactions to the Expressed Emotion Reactions of Caregivers

Criticism, hostility, and withdrawal may serve to alienate the individual with anorexia, who consequentially withdraws further into the company of the anorexic voice. They may feel misunderstood, disrespected, and ignored, resulting in a mirroring of anger; the anorexic voice does not respond to logic, and so the battle is never won.

Overprotection can promote the exclusive "sick role", which can lead to envy and/or neglect from other family members. As the individual becomes infantilized, their social and emotional development becomes atrophied because their problems are "fixed" by others. Over time, family members may seek to avoid provoking anxiety or conflict by accommodating or enabling the symptoms (Sepulveda, Kyriacou, & Treasure, 2009). In Table 7.1, the context (why) that elicits the emotionally driven behaviors (what) is described.

The Impact of Anorexia Nervosa on Social Cognition and the Indirect (Less Visible) Influence on Close Others

Aside from the overt eating disorder behaviors, many secondary symptoms have an influence on others that arise because of the consequence of starvation on the brain, with social cognition particularly impacted. In the acute state, patients have moderate to large impairments in several domains of social cognition, including facial expressivity, interpretation of non-verbal expression of others, and theory of mind (Caglar-Nazali et al., 2014). Moreover, possibly because of the state of high stress and arousal, people with anorexia nervosa have an increased sensitivity to threat and a negative bias in attention to and interpretation of social scenarios (Cardi et al., 2015; Harrison, Sullivan, Tchanturia, & Treasure, 2010). Overall, these difficulties lead to a lack of social reciprocity and a developing sense of alienation.

Reaction of Close Others to Impaired Social Cognition and Sensitivity to Threat (Less Visible) Influences

Impairments in social cognition impact on others by disrupting social communication, as if the person with the eating disorder is not speaking the same language. Starvation disrupts interoceptive processes and bodily feedback, leading to a lack of facial expressivity – a cold, aloof reaction, as if they were an "ice maiden" with a "deadpan" face (Caglar-Nazali et al., 2014; Davies et al., 2016; Leppanen et al., 2017). The absence of normal facial expressivity is disturbing and triggers feelings of disgust and dislike in others (Hess & Fischer, 2013; Schneider, Hempel, & Lynch, 2013; Szczurek, Monin, & Gross, 2012). Indeed, social interactions with people inhibiting their emotional expressions leads to physiological stress responses (increases in blood pressure) and reduces motivation to further engage socially (Butler et al., 2003). This is similar to the "uncanny valley" effect towards computer-generated images, in which people have negative emotional reactions to representations that are almost human (Ciechanowski, Przegalinska, Magnuski, & Gloor, 2018).

Alexithymia is the inability to identify and describes one's own emotions and is shown to be present in varying degrees in people with eating disorders, being elevated to a greater extent in people with anorexia, in whom this deficit extends to processing emotion in others (Lavender et al., 2015). The embodied cognition literature details how we mirror and embody the physiological emotional responses of others when empathizing and that these empathic responses can be modulated by the degree of alexithymia (Bernhardt & Singer, 2012). Indeed, social cognition, empathy, and theory of mind are impaired in anorexia (Beadle, Paradiso, Salerno, & McCormick, 2013; Harrison, Sullivan, & Tchanturia, 2015), which makes reciprocity in social interactions more difficult. Interestingly, people with anorexia show difficulty in detecting intimacy (Renwick et al., 2013).

Moreover, attention and interpretation biases to the negative further disrupt interpersonal interactions. People with anorexia nervosa are hypersensitive to threats of social exclusion, negatively interpreting social scenarios (Cardi et al., 2017), attending to rejection cues while avoiding social reward ones (Cardi et al., 2015; Cardi, Matteo, Corfield, &

Treasure, 2013; Harrison et al., 2010) and displaying less effective social problem-solving skills (Sternheim et al., 2012); these biases are linked with levels of depression, anxiety, and eating disorder symptomatology. The impact on others is that this overt sensitivity to threat leads people with anorexia to interpret and respond coldly to emotional warmth (Ambwani et al., 2016). This avoidant interpersonal and emotional processing inadvertently serves to maintain the illness' symptoms (Treasure & Schmidt, 2013).

Targeting the Interpersonal Elements of the Cognitive Interpersonal Model

In the previous section, we describe how starvation impacts on social cognition and disrupts the fine-tuning needed for successful social connection. Furthermore, the visible and socially disruptive behaviors associated with anorexia nervosa also have an impact on close others. Thus, there are two possible targets for treatment: direct by solving the starvation effects and indirect by moderating the interpersonal reactions to the illness, both in the patient and their carers. The direct approach is more effective in the early stage of the illness. However, when the illness has proved to be resistant to early phase approaches, then a more indirect approach may be of value, such as through moderating interpersonal reactions to reduce social alienation.

Therefore, carers may need to approach the problem from a meta level of understanding and modify their habitual response patterns. This formulation can seem unfair to carers and lead to counter reactions, such as "It is my daughter who needs changing, not me". We reply in line with the Viktor Frankl quote: "When we are no longer able to change a situation – we are challenged to change ourselves". We may also use the aeroplane analogy "adults need to get their own oxygen first" to emphasize the need for support and reflection.

It is understandable that caregivers are primed to behave abnormally in the abnormal situation they are in. We discuss how the cognitive interpersonal model was developed to describe the interpersonal problems that can arise on inpatient units (Treasure, Crane, Mcknight, Buchanan, & Wolfe, 2011). Indeed, the training we give carers is the same as we use to train inpatient teams; in accordance with our philosophy of collaborative practice, we often do joint training workshops.

The latest genetic findings suggest that the vulnerability to anorexia nervosa arises from both brain and metabolically expressed genes (Duncan et al., 2017; Ilyas et al., 2018), which may explain how abnormal feedback signals from the body can contribute to the ill state. This externalizes the mechanisms onto the disease itself rather than onto individuals, a useful technique to avert frustration. We are clear that the cognitive interpersonal model does not ascribe fault to carers. Rather, we use Figure 7.1 to show the complex entanglement that arises from living in close proximity to anorexia nervosa.

With carers, we have co-created the animal metaphors to take away the sting that technical terms within the model can produce and to provide an easy-to-remember prompt to break automated habits. We have termed overprotection as "Kangaroo" care, Hostility and Criticism as "Rhino" and "Terrier" approaches, and Avoidance as the "Ostrich" with its head in the sand. We do not denigrate any of these responses but emphasize that although at times they have their place, for change to occur they may need to be moderated and time limited. We use motivational interviewing techniques with readiness rulers so that carers can help each other to stay longer together in the middle ground.

Improving Communication and Support

The metaphors that we have developed to describe behaviors that we want carers to emulate and role model include the Dolphin, St Bernard, and herd of Elephants (Table 7.2).

Strategies to Moderate Maladaptive Interpersonal Reactions

In Table 7.3, we describe the theoretical rationale and the skills and strategies that can be used to reduce carers' emotionally driven behaviors. Carers are encouraged to follow a basic protocol to change their own behavior (awareness, planning, trying it, followed by reflection), which is also a template to model how to move forwards with recovery for the individual with an eating disorder. The aims are to enable carers to reflect and role model change responses. A manual describing how to implement these strategies in workshops is available (Langley, Treasure, &

Table 7.2 Caregiving behaviors to be increased

Metaphor	Description
Dolphin	This is used to summarize a wise, nudging, hands-off type of approach. To adopt this approach, we teach carers the principles of motivational interviewing. We also note the "smile" of the dolphin and suggest that they remember to use this to step aside from mirroring the by-products of starvation such as fear and anger.
St Bernard	This is used to convey the need to stay close to provide warmth and nurture to the ill individual who is lost in the frozen waste of anorexia nervosa. The St Bernard instils hope that the sufferer can change, that there is a future full of possibility beyond the eating disorder. The St Bernard responds consistently and is unfailing, reliable, and dependable in all circumstances.
Herd of Elephants	The head-to-tail connection of elephant herds is used to convey how important it is to work as a team both within the family and with health professionals. In a herd of elephants, leadership is not related to dominance; rather, it comes about through respect for others in the group and the collective ability to solve problems.

Table 7.3 Theories and strategies to moderate maladaptive interpersonal reactions

Behavior	Theoretical Rationale or Psychoeducation	Strategy Taught to Carer
General	• It is common for individuals and social networks to oscillate through the spectrum of animal responses. • Balance and flexibility are key; each type of response has its place depending on the context.	• Rating scales are used to reflect on the most common animal model or their emotional and behavioral reactions to the eating disorder (individual and interpersonal scores).
Overprotection (Kangaroo)	• Avoidance perpetuates anxiety. • Mastery and action build self-confidence. • Perfectionism is a fear of making mistakes that inhibits new learning. • Learning in the brain is facilitated by surprises. • "Every mistake is a treasure".	• Carer uses a coaching style (belief in individual) rather than a "Mr Fix It" approach to build self-efficacy. • Carer elicits decisions from the individual through offering a choice out of two options. • Carer encourages opposing emotional behaviors, such as the courage (rather than avoidance) to take safe risks. • Carer grounds the individual within the "big picture".

(Continued)

Table 7.3 (Continued)

Behavior	Theoretical Rationale or Psychoeducation	Strategy Taught to Carer
Criticism, Hostility (Rhinoceros, Terrier)	• Anorexia nervosa is influenced by genes that have an impact on the brain and metabolism. • Difficulty getting out from weight loss trap.	• Empathetic coaching: plan, do, and reflect cycles for change; small manageable steps to set goals. • Negotiate the form and content of support. • Carer develops compassion and positively reframes negative reactions.
Avoidance (Ostrich)	• Strength in social network. • Fathers and other partners can play a key role in recovery.	• Solution-focused strategies to provide balance. • Develop simple risk-taking experiments to shift avoidant position.

Accommodation and enabling	• Awareness.
	• It is easier to change your own behavior than that of other people.
	• Carers modeling behavior change can be an example for the offspring.
		• Use of accommodation and enabling questionnaire to highlight how these behaviors are common and pervasive (Sepulveda et al., 2009).
		• Teach behavior change strategies:
		  • Motivation: pros and cons of change
		  • Ability: small steps; make careful plans and enlist the help of others
		  • Trigger: prepare, share, and reflect on plans in calm time
		  • Strategies of nonviolent resistance such as used in childhood obsessive-compulsive disorder and anxiety may be of value (Lebowitz & Omer, 2013).

Fragmentation	• Teaching that counterbalancing extreme behaviors (e.g. increasing overprotection to oppose hostility in others harms rather than helps. • Inconsistent accommodating behaviors "fix" anorexia behaviors and produce "splitting".	• Co-operative planning for a shared approach. • Aim for a united response around the middle ground. Practice accepting "good enough" solutions.

Todd, 2018), as is a manual for carers themselves (Treasure, Smith, & Crane, 2016). Both have co-authorship between people with lived experience and professionals.

What Is the Effectiveness of Skill-Sharing Interventions?

Training carers with the skills to sidestep unhelpful interactions and to reduce the isolation of anorexia nervosa is of benefit, both in terms of carer distress and effort and for patient wellbeing. For example, providing carers of inpatients with self-management tools reduced length of stay and readmission in the six months after discharge (Hibbs et al., 2015), and small improvements in patient symptoms were observed (with a small effect size) two years later (Magill et al., 2016). Moreover, these interventions reduced carers' expressed emotion and time spent caring. A similar pattern of improvements was attained by augmenting treatment as usual with the carer intervention ECHO (Experienced Carers Helping Others); again, there were lower admission rates and improved psychosocial functioning in both adolescents and their carers (Hodsoll et al., 2017). A pilot study has found that a hybrid intervention ECHO MANTRA with modules for both patients and carers has the potential to improve transitions from inpatient care (Adamson et al., 2019).

Conclusion

The cognitive interpersonal model explains the domino effect from anorexia nervosa that causes it to become a chronic illness resistant to treatment. This model highlights how it is possible to cut through this Gordian knot and use compassionate leverage to move towards change. Maximizing social support by changing automatic reactions to the illness by any individuals in the caring role can moderate outcomes that are relevant for the patient and promote recovery.

Acknowledgments

We would like to acknowledge and thank all the patients and carers over the years who have contributed to research to help us better understand the illness to inform treatment development. We would also like to acknowledge financial support from the National Institute for Health Research (NIHR) Specialist Biomedical Research Centre for Mental Health award to the South London and Maudsley NHS Foundation Trust and the Institute of Psychiatry, King's College London.

References

Adamson, J., Cardi, V., Kan, C., Harrison, A., Macdonald, P., & Treasure, J. (2019). Evaluation of a novel transition support intervention in an adult eating disorders service: ECHOMANTRA. *International Review of Psychiatry*, 1–9.

Ambwani, S., Berenson, K. R., Simms, L., Li, A., Corfield, F., & Treasure, J. (2016). Seeing things differently: An experimental investigation of social cognition and interpersonal behavior in anorexia nervosa. *International Journal of Eating Disorders*, *49*(5), 499–506. https://doi.org/10.1002/eat.22498

Anastasiadou, D., Medina-Pradas, C., Sepulveda, A. R., & Treasure, J. (2014). A systematic review of family caregiving in eating disorders. *Eating Behaviors*, *15*(3), 464–477.

Beadle, J. N., Paradiso, S., Salerno, A., & McCormick, L. M. (2013). Alexithymia, emotional empathy, and self-regulation in anorexia nervosa. *Annals of Clinical Psychiatry*, *25*(2), 107–120. https://doi.org/10.1007/s11103-011-9767-z.Plastid

Bernhardt, B. C., & Singer, T. (2012). The neural basis of empathy. *Annual Review of Neuroscience*, *35*(1), 1–23. https://doi.org/10.1146/annurev-neuro-062111-150536

Butler, E. A., Egloff, B., Wilhelm, F. H., Smith, N. C., Erickson, E. A., & Gross, J. J. (2003). The social consequences of expressive suppression. *Emotion*, *3*(1), 48–67. https://doi.org/10.1037/1528-3542.3.1.48

Caglar-Nazali, H. P., Corfield, F., Cardi, V., Ambwani, S., Leppanen, J., Olabintan, O., . . . Treasure, J. (2014). A systematic review and meta-analysis of "systems for social processes" in eating disorders. *Neuroscience and Biobehavioral Reviews*, *42*, 55–92. https://doi.org/10.1016/j.neubiorev.2013.12.002

Cardi, V., Esposito, M., Bird, G., Rhind, C., Yiend, J., Schifano, S., . . . Treasure, J. (2015). A preliminary investigation of a novel training to target cognitive biases towards negative social stimuli in anorexia nervosa. *Journal of Affective Disorders*, *188*, 188–193. https://doi.org/http://dx.doi.org/10.1016/j.jad.2015.08.019

Cardi, V., Matteo, R. D., Corfield, F., & Treasure, J. (2013). Social reward and rejection sensitivity in eating disorders: An investigation of attentional bias and early experiences. *World Journal of Biological Psychiatry*, *14*(8), 622–633. https://doi.org/10.3109/15622975.2012.665479

Cardi, V., Turton, R., Schifano, S., Leppanen, J., Hirsch, C. R., & Treasure, J. (2017). Biased interpretation of ambiguous social scenarios in anorexia nervosa. *European Eating Disorders Review*, *25*(1), 60–64. https://doi.org/10.1002/erv.2493

Ciechanowski, L., Przegalinska, A., Magnuski, M., & Gloor, P. (2018). In the shades of the uncanny valley: An experimental study of human-chatbot interaction. *Future Generation Computer Systems*, *92*, 539–548. https://doi.org/10.1016/j.future.2018.01.055

Davies, H., Wolz, I., Leppanen, J., Fernandez-Aranda, F., Schmidt, U., & Tchanturia, K. (2016). Facial expression to emotional stimuli in non-psychotic disorders: A systematic review and meta-analysis. *Neuroscience & Biobehavioral Reviews*, *64*, 252–271.

Duncan, L., Yilmaz, Z., Gaspar, H., Walters, R., Goldstein, J., Anttila, V., . . . Ripke, S. (2017). Significant locus and metabolic genetic correlations revealed in genome-wide association study of anorexia nervosa. *American Journal of Psychiatry*, *174*(9), 850–858. https://doi.org/10.1176/appi.ajp.2017.16121402

Eisler, I., Dare, C., Russell, G. F., Szmukler, G., Le Grange, D., & Dodge, E. (1997). Family and individual therapy in anorexia nervosa: A 5-year follow-up. *Archives of General Psychiatry*, *54*(11), 1025–1030. https://doi.org/10.1037/14295-017

Haigh, R., & Treasure, J. (2003). Investigating the needs of carers in the area of eating disorders: Development of the Carers' Needs Assessment Measure (CaNAM). *European Eating Disorders Review*, *11*(2), 125–141. https://doi.org/10.1002/erv.487

Harrison, A., Mountford, V. A., & Tchanturia, K. (2014). Social anhedonia and work and social functioning in the acute and recovered phases of eating disorders. *Psychiatry Research*, *218*(1–2), 187–194. https://doi.org/10.1016/j.psychres.2014.04.007

Harrison, A., Sullivan, S., & Tchanturia, K. (2015, October). Emotion recognition and regulation in anorexia emotion recognition and regulation in anorexia nervosa. *356*, 348–356. https://doi.org/10.1002/cpp.628

Harrison, A., Sullivan, S., Tchanturia, K., & Treasure, J. (2010). Emotional functioning in eating disorders: Attentional bias, emotion recognition and emotion regulation. *Psychological Medicine*, *40*(11), 1887–1897. https://doi.org/10.1017/S0033291710000036

Hess, U., & Fischer, A. (2013). Emotional mimicry as social regulation. *Personality and Social Psychology Review*, *17*(2), 142–157. https://doi.org/10.1177/1088868312472607

Hibbs, R., Magill, N., Goddard, E., Rhind, C., Raenker, S., Macdonald, P., . . . Treasure, J. (2015). Clinical effectiveness of a skills training intervention for caregivers in improving patient and caregiver health following in-patient treatment for severe anorexia nervosa: Pragmatic randomised controlled trial. *British Journal of Psychiatry Open*, *1*(1), 56–66. https://doi.org/10.1192/bjpo.bp.115.000273

Hodsoll, J., Rhind, C., Micali, N., Hibbs, R., Goddard, E., Nazar, B. P., . . . Treasure, J. (2017). A pilot, multicentre pragmatic randomised trial to explore the impact of carer skills training on carer and patient behaviours: Testing the cognitive interpersonal model in adolescent anorexia nervosa. *European Eating Disorders Review*, *25*(6), 551–561. https://doi.org/10.1002/erv.2540

Ilyas, A., Hübel, C., Stahl, D., Stadler, M., Ismail, K., Breen, G., . . . Kan, C. (2018, October). Molecular and cellular endocrinology the metabolic underpinning of eating disorders: A systematic review and meta-analysis of insulin sensitivity. *Molecular and Cellular Endocrinology*, 1–8. https://doi.org/10.1016/j.mce.2018.10.005

Kyriacou, O., Treasure, J., & Schmidt, U. (2008). Expressed emotion in eating disorders assessed via self-report: An examination of factors associated with expressed emotion in carers of people with anorexia nervosa in comparison to control families. *International Journal of Eating Disorders*, *41*(1), 37–46. Retrieved from https://onlinelibrary.wiley.com/doi/epdf/10.1002/eat.20469

Langley, J., Treasure, J., & Todd, G. (2018). *Caring for a loved one with an eating disorder: The new Maudsley skills-based training manual*. London: Routledge.

Lavender, J. M., Wonderlich, S. A., Engel, S. G., Gordon, K. H., Kaye, W. H., & Mitchell, J. E. (2015). Dimensions of emotion dysregulation in anorexia nervosa and bulimia nervosa: A conceptual review of the empirical literature. *Clinical Psychology Review*, *40*, 111–122. https://doi.org/10.1016/j.cpr.2015.05.010

Lebowitz, E., & Omer, H. (2013). *Treating childhood and adolescent anxiety: A guide for caregivers*. Hoboken, NJ: John Wiley & Sons.

Lebowitz, E. R., Panza, K. E., & Bloch, M. H. (2016). Family accommodation in obsessive-compulsive and anxiety disorders: A five-year update. *Expert Review of Neurotherapeutics*, *16*(1), 45–53.

Leppanen, J., Dapelo, M.M., Davies, H., Lang, K., Treasure, J., Tchanturia, K. (2017) Computerised analysis of facial emotion expression in eating disorders. *PLoS One*, *12*(6), e0178972

Levine, M. P. (2012). Loneliness and eating disorders. *Journal of Psychology: Interdisciplinary and Applied*, *146*(1–2), 243–257. https://doi.org/10.1080/00223980.2011.606435

Magill, N., Rhind, C., Hibbs, R., Goddard, E., Macdonald, P., Arcelus, J., . . . Treasure, J. (2016). Two-year follow-up of a pragmatic randomised controlled trial examining the effect of adding a carer's skill training intervention in inpatients with anorexia nervosa. *European Eating Disorders Review*, *24*(2), 122–130. https://doi.org/10.1002/erv.2422

McKnight, R., & Boughton, N. (2014). Anorexia nervosa. *British Medical Journal*, *22*(2), 1–9.

Renwick, B., Dejong, H., Kenyon, M., Samarawickrema, N., Loomes, R., Watson, C., . . . Schmidt, U. (2013). Social perception in people with eating disorders. *European Psychiatry*, *28*(7), 436–441. https://doi.org/10.1016/j.eurpsy.2013.03.004

Russell, G. F., Szmukler, G., Dare, C., & Eisler, I. (1987). An evaluation of family therapy in anorexia nervosa and bulimia nervosa. *Archives of General Psychiatry*, *44*(12), 1047–1056. Retrieved from http://cochranelibrary-wiley.com/o/cochrane/clcentral/articles/277/CN-00051277/frame.html

Schmidt, U., & Treasure, J. (2006). Anorexia nervosa: Valued and visible: A cognitive-interpersonal maintenance model and its implications for research and practice. *British Journal of Clinical Psychology*, *45*(3), 343–366. https://doi.org/10.1348/014466505X53902

Schneider, K. G., Hempel, R. J., & Lynch, T. R. (2013). That "poker face" just might lose you the game! the impact of expressive suppression and mimicry on sensitivity to facial expressions of emotion. *Emotion*, *13*(5), 852–866. https://doi.org/10.1037/a0032847

Sepulveda, A. R., Kyriacou, O., & Treasure, J. (2009). Development and validation of the Accommodation and Enabling Scale for Eating Disorders (AESED) for caregivers in eating disorders. *BMC Health Services Research*, *9*, 1–13. https://doi.org/10.1186/1472-6963-9-171

Sternheim, L., Startup, H., Pretorius, N., Johnson-sabine, E., Schmidt, U., & Channon, S. (2012). An experimental exploration of social problem solving and its associated processes in anorexia nervosa. *Psychiatry Research*, *200*(2–3), 524–529. https://doi.org/10.1016/j.psychres.2012.06.029

Szczurek, L., Monin, B., & Gross, J. J. (2012). The stranger effect: The rejection of affective deviants. *Psychological Science*, *23*(10), 1105–1111. https://doi.org/10.1177/0956797612445314

Treasure, J., Crane, A., Mcknight, R., Buchanan, E., & Wolfe, M. (2011). First do no harm: Iatrogenic maintaining factors in anorexia nervosa. *European Eating Disorders Review*, *19*, 296–302. https://doi.org/10.1002/erv.1056

Treasure, J., & Schmidt, U. (2013). The cognitive-interpersonal maintenance model of anorexia nervosa revisited: A summary of the evidence for cognitive, socio-emotional and interpersonal predisposing and perpetuating factors. *Journal of Eating Disorders*, *1*(1), 1–10. https://doi.org/10.1186/2050-2974-1-13

Treasure, J., Smith, G., & Crane, A. (2016). *Skills-based caring for a loved one with an eating disorder: The new Maudsley method*. London: Routledge.

Whitney, J., Murray, J., Gavan, K., Todd, G., Whitaker, W., & Treasure, J. (2005). Experience of caring for someone with anorexia nervosa: Qualitative study. *British Journal of Psychiatry*, *187*, 444–449. https://doi.org/10.1192/bjp.187.5.444

8

Cultural Differences in Expressed Emotion

Tecelli Domínguez-Martínez and Cristina Medina-Pradas

Introduction

Culture can be defined as shared patterns of behaviors and interactions, cognitive constructs, and understanding that individuals learn and dynamically create and recreate for themselves in the process of socialization (Shweder & LeVine, 1984). Psychological anthropologists have shown that emotions, attitudes, beliefs, and behaviors can no longer properly be considered a private, intrapsychic, or psychobiological phenomenon because these are substantially mediated by culture (e.g., Jenkins, Karno, de la Selva, & Santana, 1986; Jenkins & Karno, 1992). A culture also offers models of how people should or may feel and act in response to the serious mental illness of a loved one. This may involve anger and hostility in one context or sadness and sympathy in another (Jenkins & Karno, 1992).

The Expressed Emotion (EE) Index (Leff & Vaughn, 1985) is regarded as measuring cultural features because it taps a set of shared meanings and patterns of affective response to the problem of living with mental illness in a family environment. The nature and meaning of EE components are understood to be culturally specific, because culture determines whether any type of EE is a prominent part of the emotional response among family members, the specific content or target of various EE components, and the factors influencing their levels (Jenkins & Karno, 1992; Cheng, 2002). Thus, EE research requires a cross-cultural perspective to better explain the development of this construct in different populations, as well as differences in its constructs depending on cultural context (Jenkins & Karno, 1992; Medina-Pradas, Navarro, Pousa, Montero, & Obiols, 2013; Mottaghipour, Pourmand, Maleki, & Davidian, 2001; Cheng, 2002; Bhugra & McKenzie, 2003; López et al., 2009; Scherer, Clark-Polner, & Mortillaro, 2011).

Cultural Variability in Expressed Emotion

The study of EE was initially focused on Anglo-Saxon families of patients with schizophrenia (e.g., Brown, 1985; Kuipers, 1987; Vaughn, 1989). The anthropological and cross-cultural psychiatric literature of the past several decades has documented substantial cultural differences in conceptions and features that are key for the understanding of EE, such as display of emotion, family structure, and behavioral rules and norms (Jenkins & Karno, 1992). As a consequence, research in the field of EE has been gradually increasing and applied to a variety of both psychiatric and nonpsychiatric conditions in different populations worldwide (Wearden, Tarrier, & Barrowclough, 2000). A family's EE has been shown to be predictive of outcome in mental and physical illnesses in a variety of cultural settings (Bhugra & McKenzie, 2003). Evidence of research on EE across different national and ethnic groups suggests that the sociocultural context may influence the family's emotional climate and the levels of EE. The distribution and mean scores of Criticism, Hostility, and Emotional Overinvolvement (EOI) are also significantly different across cultures (Leff & Vaughn, 1985; López et al., 2009; Bhugra & McKenzie, 2003).

Although verbal criticism within families is likely to occur in most of the world's cultures, there is a cross-cultural variation in the frequency, intensity, nature, and meaning of criticism within families (Jenkins & Karno, 1992). For example, within Anglo-American family settings, criticism may focus on allegations of faulty personality traits (e.g., laziness) or psychotic symptom behaviors (e.g., strange ideas), while the same behaviors may not be met with criticism among Mexican descent families, who tend to focus on disrespectful or disruptive behaviors that affect the family instead of on the symptoms or behaviors and individual personality characteristics (Jenkins et al., 1986; Jenkins & Karno, 1992). Moreover, Kamal (1995) reported that Egyptian patients tolerated higher levels of criticism before relapse than those which have been reported in Western studies. It has been suggested that criticism is an accepted component of interpersonal relations in Egyptian culture and that it might well reflect an element of care or benign criticism (Kamal, 1995; Okasha et al., 1994). Comparison between Japanese and English samples showed a greater number of Critical Comments in English relatives. This could be explained by the fact that in Japanese culture, individuals tend to be reserved in displaying their emotions in public and reluctant to overtly criticize their relatives. This probably affects a broad spectrum of EE responses in the Japanese samples (Nomura et al., 2005). Studies in Israel have demonstrated that anger is more openly and more immediately expressed than in Western countries, because failure to express one's anger is perceived as a weakness. Thus, it is likely that both Hostility and Critical Comments seen in the context of Israelis may result in false-positive rates of high expressed emotion (Heresco-Levy, Greenberg, & Dasberg, 1990).

EOI is seen in the West as pathological because it crosses the boundaries of individuals, whereas in some parts of India, it is not necessarily pathological but is the norm, that is, if a carer does not show EOI, it is seen as a lack of care. Similarly, in Jewish settings, mothers' Critical Comments and EOI are culture related and should not be perceived as pathological (Bhugra & McKenzie, 2003). Ethnic differences on EE components have also been found between the Mexican-American and Anglo-American samples. Lopez's team in California (U.S.A.), for instance, who has investigated this issue in schizophrenia, has repeatedly found that the Mexican-American sample expressed a significantly lower number of Critical Comments, less Hostility, more EOI, and more Warmth than did the Anglo-American sample (Kopelowicz et al., 2002; López et al., 2009). They also found that high-EE only predicted relapse for Anglo Americans. This is consistent with previous studies showing that Mexican-American caregivers tend to express considerable empathy for the condition of their ill relatives (instead of judge them) and are more involved in the lives of their ill relatives than Anglo-American family caregivers (Weisman, López, Karno, & Jenkins, 1993; Ramírez-García, Wood, Hosch, & Meyer, 2004; Snowden, 2007). These findings highlight the importance of taking greater attention in the study of EOI, at least among primarily immigrant Mexican Americans and other culture groups that promote high degree of involvement with ill relatives (Jenkins & Karno, 1992; López et al., 2009).

Similar conclusions have been reached by Weisman de Mamani, Kymalainen, Rosales, and Armesto (2007), and Kymalainen, Weisman, Rosales, and Armesto (2006). Latino family members of patients with schizophrenia living in a family-oriented culture, in which values are placed on collectivism and interdependence, have been found to show lower rates of high EE than white and black families, as examples of more autonomous cultures in which values are placed on independence and personal goal achievement. Finally, in the review of Kymalainen and Weisman (2008), it was proposed that more attention should be paid to the role of cultural values and norms and the impact of their violation on the family–patient relationship. Moreover, in dementia, Connell and Gibson (1997) reviewed 12 studies and concluded that non-white caregivers exhibited lower levels of stress, burden, and depression than white caregivers.

In addition to comparisons between whites versus ethnic minorities in a specific location, other ways of cultural comparisons can be considered in a cross-cultural analysis. In this sense, criteria like individualistic (f.i. Western) versus collectivistic (f.i. China) societies would be considered (Cha, 1994; Nagayama Hall, 2001). Cheng (2002) suggested some interesting differences concerning EE in this regard. When comparing studies with schizophrenia patients in Chinese families, in which obedience and acceptance of parental criticism are encouraged, carers manifested higher levels of EE than Western families, in which autonomy, pursuit of personal goals, and equality among family members are emphasized.

Moreover, in a sample of African-American and Hispanic carers of patients with cancer, it was concluded that the caregiving experience may be independent of race or ethnicity and that sociodemographic variables may have a greater impact on this experience than culture-related variables (Siefert, Williams, Dowd, Chappel-Aiken, & McCorkle., 2008).

Evidence shows that prevalence of high-EE families tended to be lower in non-Western countries than in Western countries (Bhugra & McKenzie, 2003; Kymalainen & Weisman de Mamani, 2008). However, in some Western countries, such as Italy and Spain, EE was lower than in the U.S.A. or England (Kavanagh, 1992; Meneghelli et al., 2011). It has been suggested that EE may be a measure of the meaning that relatives attribute to behaviors, which are perceived as violating culturally endorsed social norms. For example, white Anglo Saxons place primary emphasis on independence, and some symptoms of schizophrenia might violate family members' expectations of patients' autonomy and independence (Jenkins & Karno, 1992). In contrast, other cultural groups put greater emphasis on the values associated with family unity, interdependence, and the sense of interconnectedness with others and therefore would be less likely to blame their relatives for symptoms of illness to preserve family cohesion, resulting in lower EE (Weisman, 2005; Singelis, 1994). Also, in Mediterranean countries, EOI overlaps with the more emotional implication typical of those cultures (Medina-Pradas, Navarro, López, Grau, & Obiols, 2011a; Domínguez-Martínez, Medina-Pradas, Kwapil, & Barrantes-Vidal, 2014, 2017), and some authors have even suggested to change the cut-off point for high EOI in this respect (Bertrando et al., 1992).

Additionally, it is important to consider that changes in levels of EE may be influenced by processes of acculturation (the psychological, behavioral, and attitudinal changes that occur through cultural exchange and contact with different social groups) if cultural groups move across national and cultural boundaries (Heresco-Levy et al., 1990). In a sample of 60 Mexican-American caregivers and their ill relatives, Aguilera, López, Breitborde, Kopelowicz, and Zarate (2010) found that acculturation and enculturation (the process of preserving own language use and cultural norms) moderate the relationship between EE and clinical outcomes.

The understanding of EE through a cross-cultural perspective can contribute to a reflective understanding based less on an assumption of autonomous sentiments and actions and more on a constellation of shared features (Lefley, 1987). However, some important limitations to existing culturally focused research should be considered. A focus on global EE may limit the identification of sociocultural influences on specific family processes (Aguilera et al., 2010). Thus, a more complete and better assessment of cross-cultural differences would be to examine high-EE profiles as well as the distributions of specific EE ratings across the entire sample (López et al., 2009). Furthermore, cultural variation in the degree and type of EE must be studied carefully and well understood to apply the principles of EE across different cultural groups and settings. If EE represents the "emotional temperature" of a person or family, researchers must first establish the "normal" temperature of families from a cultural group before determining which temperature higher than that norm is pathological (Singh, Harley, & Suhail, 2013). Besides, the cross-cultural validity of EE factors requires close attention to the autochthonous definitions and expressions of Criticism, Hostility, and EOI (Jenkins, 1991).

The focus on specific EE indices begins to suggest how culture may shape the relationship of family factors and course of illness. However, the focus on relapse as the main outcome measure may restrict our understanding of how family factors and culture influence the course of illness (Aguilera et al., 2010).

The study of nationality and ethnicity is an important first step to identify the role of culture in the EE-clinical course relationship, but culture should be consider as a process rather than a category. In addition, the use of more direct and proxy measures of culture such as place of birth (foreign born versus native born), language dominance (Spanish or English), and acculturation level could also serve to buttress cultural interpretations of cross-cultural findings and strengthen the cultural explanation (López et al., 2009; Aguilera et al., 2010).

Another limitation in the study of EE across cultures is that the original EE indices and their ratings often require some adaptation to the specific cultural context (e.g., Jenkins, 1991; Phillips & Xiong, 1995; López et al., 2009). Given that original measures of EE were created based on the Anglo-Saxon context (especially the Camberwell Family Interview), what is considered a normative degree of family emotions for British, Americans, or Australians, it could result in over-identification or false-positive rates of EE in another cultural context or vice versa. Thus, the observed cross-ethnic or cross-national differences may not necessarily reflect cultural differences in EE but instead may reflect the incongruities of the non-adapted measure when applied in a new cultural context (López et al., 2009). It should be noted that all researchers make at least some modifications to the new cultural context, particularly when the measures are translated from English into another language. However, there are potential limitations in adapting the original rating scale, because modifying the metric makes it difficult to compare the findings with other studies that make little or no adjustments. The literature is not clear about when and how cultural adjustments should be made, but in cases that adjustments are made, it is important to document specifically how such modifications were carried out, as well as to test whether the culturally adjusted EE domain measures have incremental predictive validity compared with the unadjusted measure (López et al., 2009).

Several studies have emphasized the importance of considering and understanding cultural norms in the measurement and rating of EE, especially when the interviewer does not belong to the cultural group of the respondent. EE ratings must be adjusted in relation to the normative levels of overt expression of emotions, which vary across cultures (Heresco-Levy et al., 1990; Bhugra & McKenzie, 2003). The levels and the prevalence of the various components of the rating scale also vary. For example, tone of voice can play a role in the identification of high EE, but in several cultures, speaking loudly is the norm (Jenkins & Karno, 1992). Studies with Japanese and Chinese samples have shown that it is highly likely that the people who speak Asian languages require more time to reach the point of their criticism and may be more reticent and indirect in criticizing the patient compared with English relatives, reflecting significant differences in terms of communication style that exist between East and West (Kaplan, 1966). Furthermore, Asian respondents may be reluctant to overtly criticize relatives with whom they have a specific relationship determined by social structure, such as their parents. Moreover, Mottaghipour et al. (2001) found that in an Iranian sample, Hostility was the most common component of EE contributing to a high overall rating, instead of Critical Comments, as has been reported in previous studies in general or EOI in Mediterranean studies. By analyzing the context, authors suggest that according to Iranian culture, during the interview relatives probably mentioned negative aspects and emphasized complaints as a way of asking for all the help they could get from mental health services. In contrast, it has been shown that relatives in some cultures tend to mask their negative attitudes and emotional responses in front of interviewers (Phillips & Xiong, 1995). Thus, future research also needs to explore whether the measure of EE, mainly used in Western cultures, has universal utility in investigating clinical populations in Eastern cultures (Nomura et al., 2005).

Given that it is difficult for a researcher to rate any of the components of EE when he or she is not familiar with the nuances of language and cultural expression of an interviewee, measurement of EE should be carried out by a person from the same cultural group of the respondents. Further, if measures of EE are being applied in cultures in which they have not been used before, they must be accompanied by fieldwork to establish the norms and the context. The most important factor for the researcher is to embed EOI, Hostility, and Warmth in the specific cultural context. Measurement is also dependent on an assessment of the interviewee's general style of EE (Bhugra & McKenzie, 2003).

Furthermore, raters assessing EE by interview in different cultures might be influenced by their own non-Western cultural backgrounds. Thus, more studies of cross-cultural validity and inter-rater reliability are required, in which researchers from different cultures observe, use EE measures, and rate relatives' EE of individuals and families from different cultures. This could establish the differences in content, meaning, expression, and cultural norms of any EE observed by any rater. Similarly, it is important to consider the possible influence on EE assessment of differences in the frequency of contact between patients and relatives, the types of relatives, and the impact of interviewer and interview context on the respondents (Cheng, 2002).

Cross-Cultural Aspects of Eating Disorders

In most cultures, eating is a habit with a social value that varies widely between religious and ethnic groups. Eating socialization, culinary traditions, eating patterns, prescribed dietary norms, and attitudes toward food are established by an individual's culture and are primarily learned within a familial context (Birch & Fisher, 1998; Haworth-Hoeppner, 2000). Thus, understanding culture (individuals' experiences as members of a larger social group and their values and beliefs) and its influence on eating habits is essential to the comprehension of the etiology and development of eating pathology (Markey, 2004; Keel & Klump, 2003).

The increased prevalence of eating disorders (EDs) has been repeatedly shown to be a consequence of the cultivation of the ideal body, promotion of thinness values in fashion, media, and the diet industry, as well as of the social pressure resulting from the Western cultural beauty ideals for women. There is also a correlation between ED and the level of modernization and urbanization characteristic of Western industrialized societies, linking it to increased social mobility and dietary changes as well as changes within family structures (Miller & Pumariega, 2001; Nasser, 2009).

EDs were initially thought to be exclusively linked to "Western culture-bound syndrome" due to the low prevalence of these disorders in non-Western societies (Miller & Pumariega, 2001; Wildes, Emery, & Simons, 2001; Soh & Walter, 2013). Although most published research is based on North American and European populations, the notion of the culture specificity of ED began to be challenged following reports from different parts of the world where typical presentations with weight and shape-related preoccupations and fear of gaining weight had also been recorded in most non-Western cultures, including low-income countries and countries undergoing sociocultural transitions (e.g., Spain, South Africa, Mexico, India, Fiji, China, Hong Kong, Singapore, Thailand, and Japan) (Becker, Eddy, & Perloe, 2009; Lee, Lee, Ngai, Lee, & Wing, 2001; Lee, Kwok, Liau, & Leung, 2002; Al-Adawi et al., 2002; Soh & Walter, 2013). In fact, there is growing evidence that EDs are not restricted to any particular ethnic, racial, or cultural group (Winkleby, Gardener, & Taylor, 1996), but there is a repeated debate in research that EDs may present differently in patients with a non-Western background due to factors such as differing cultural values, family structure, body composition, and family environment (Soh, Touyz, & Surgenor, 2006). Research focused on immigrants to a new culture also suggests that acculturation is an important factor to consider for understanding relations between culture and eating problems (Nasser & Katzman, 1999).

Increasing globalization, the experience and exposure to the differences between two cultures (i.e., clash between a traditional culture and adopted culture), and exposure to Western culture and over-identification with Western norms and values have been hypothesized to contribute to the etiology, manifestation, and the increase of rate and incidence of EDs (Bhugra, Bhui, & Gupta, 2000; Thomas, James, & Bachmann, 2002; Lee, Ng, Kwok, & Fung, 2010; Eddy, Hennessey, & Thompson-Brenner, 2007). For example, in the Czech Republic, the incidence of anorexia nervosa (AN) increased sharply with exposure to Western-style media and values after the fall of the Iron Curtain (Pavlova, Uher, Dragomirecka, & Papezova, 2010). Further, AN is relatively rare among black women in Africa, the Caribbean, and the U.S.A. (Hoek, 2006; Njenga & Kangethe, 2004; Striegel-Moore et al., 2003). In the Caribbean island of Curaçao, all identified cases of AN were among young women of mixed ethnicity who had spent time in the U.S.A. or the Netherlands (Katzman et al., 2004; Hoek et al., 2005).

Bulimia nervosa (BN) has also been conceptualized as strongly bound to Western culture and related with the degree of acculturation (Pavlova et al., 2010; Eddy et al., 2007; Lee et al., 2010; Becker, Burwell, Herzog, Hamburg, & Gilman, 2002; Keel & Klump, 2003; Pavlova et al., 2010; Eddy et al., 2007; Al-Adawi et al., 2002; Tsai, 2000; Bhugra, Mastrogianni, Maharajh, & Harvey, 2003). Therefore, the manifestation of BN and its separation from normality needs to be considered within a cultural context. For example, culturally sanctioned feasting followed by using indigenous purgatives in Pacific Islands should not be medicalized, but the use of the same herbal purgatives in the context of typical psychopathology and outside the culturally sanctioned events is a symptom of an ED (Becker, Franko, Speck, & Herzog, 2003; Thomas et al., 2011). It has been shown that the motives for pursuing a thin body shape may also depend on socioeconomic context. For example, in societies undergoing socioeconomic transition, a thin body can be perceived as a valuable commodity that may help obtain a lucrative job and guarantee career success (Becker, 2007; Anderson-Fye, 2004; Pavlova, Uher, & Papezova, 2008).

In general, binge eating disorder (BED) and its association with obesity, weight, and shape dissatisfaction is relatively equally distributed across countries and ethnic groups, but details of manifestation vary depending on cultures (Franko, Becker, Thomas, & Herzog, 2007). Findings of a study comparing black and white women with BED found that black women are on average heavier; have fewer concerns related to body weight, shape, and eating; and have a less frequent history of BN than white women with the same diagnosis (Pike, Dohm, Striegel-Moore, Wilfley, & Fairburn, 2001).

Contrary to the widely held belief that symptoms of EDs are more pronounced in samples influenced by Western ideals of body shape, Podar and Allik (2009) in a cross-cultural comparison of the Eating Disorder

Inventory (EDI), found that non-Western participants scored higher than Western participants on most EDI subscales. Evidence in literature suggests that the prevalence of ED in non-Western groups is on the rise, but this may merely reflect growing awareness and identification of these disorders in these populations (Makino, Tsuboi, & Dennerstein, 2004; Becker, 2007). Furthermore, it is possible that the prevalence of ED in non-Western groups has been underestimated because diagnostic criteria based on Western norms may not always be appropriate to them, together with the frequent failure of health professionals to identify ED in these populations (Gordon, Perez, & Joiner, 2002; Makino et al., 2004). EDs may present differently in different racial or ethnic and national groups, and they also change across time as cultures evolve (Miller & Pumariega, 2001). However, epidemiological studies in this field are limited, and more research is needed to understand contradictions in findings in this regard.

In addition to Westernization, it is important to consider other aspects that affect the increase of ED, including cultural differences in family environment, the encroaching similarity of socioeconomic levels, consumerism, shift from collectivist to individualist patterns, changing gender roles, and increased alienation of the individual that force the individual to resort to the "body" as a new medium for expressing this cultural confusion and distress. EDs are an example of such socio-pathology and need to be seen now as a marker of "transition" and symptomatic of cultures caught in a process of change (Miller & Pumariega, 2001; Soh et al., 2006; Nasser, 2009).

Considering that health and illness are socially and culturally constructed, Markey (2004) proposes a tripartite model to better understand how cultural processes influence EDs: (1) the intergenerational transmission of dietary patterns, including food preferences and restrictive practices, may lead to the adoption of healthy and unhealthy eating behaviors; (2) values regarding physical appearance are in part culturally determined and influence eating-disordered behaviors; and (3) symptoms of ED are present among diverse populations and therefore culture influences the etiology and meaning of these symptoms.

Despite recognition of the key role of culture in the ED behavior and the apparent increase of ED in non-Western groups, there has been relatively little research published on EDs across cultures (Soh et al., 2006; Makino et al., 2004; Podarn & Allik, 2009; Soh & Walter, 2013). Most of the studies on EDs in non-Western subjects have been carried out in Western nations instead of the country of origin, without considering the degree to which an individual absorbed the mainstream Western society's values or had retained their traditional cultural values. Few studies have measured the level of acculturation, and the methods used have not been consistent across the literature. Further, few studies have been conducted in both Western and non-Western countries using the same assessment tools or did not have a sufficiently large set of cultures (Gilbert, 2003; Soh et al., 2006; Podar & Allik, 2009). Additionally, studies of EDs in non-Western cultural groups have focused mainly on African Americans, and results from such research cannot necessarily be applied to other non-Western populations (Soh & Walter, 2013).

The increasing prevalence or identification of ED in non-Western populations and the low numbers of research studies published in these population groups indicate a need to increase and expand research in this field (Soh & Walter, 2013). Further research is needed to elucidate the influence of specific cultural aspects (including protective factors) in the development of maladaptive eating behaviors and the potential causal relations across time (Markey, 2004).

Improving the understanding of the role of culture in the development of EDs can be useful for the development and delivery of culturally appropriate and acceptable treatments for individuals with EDs from diverse cultural backgrounds (Miller & Pumariega, 2001; Soh & Walter, 2013). Preventive interventions could be focused on the strengthening and/or reinforcement of ethnic identity, adaptive traditional cultural beliefs and practices, especially those that enhance self-esteem and self-concept. It would be also important that mental health professionals provide clinical care considering and respecting the patient's traditional cultural beliefs (Pumariega & Cross, 1997).

Cultural Differences of Expressed Emotion in Eating Disorders

Studies have shown that caregivers of individuals with ED experience high levels of distress, burden, and EE (Fox, Dean, & Whittlesea, 2017). Recent theoretical models have underscored the importance of caregivers' responses as a maintenance factor for the ED (Goddard et al., 2011; Treasure & Schmidt, 2013) and the effectiveness of family therapy (Gutierrez, Sepulveda, Anastasiadou, & Medina-Pradas, 2014; Treasure & Nazar, 2016).

How cultural and ethnic background influences the way in which family members interact in the context of an ED is considered crucial, but this perspective has been rarely included in research studies. Duclos, Vibert, Mattar, and Godart (2012) reviewed the literature about EE in families of patients with ED and concluded that the cross-cultural aspects of EE in ED are not widely documented. In fact, in comparison with EDs, as seen before, considerably more research related to cultural variability of EE has been conducted on family caregivers of patients with other illnesses.

Hoste, Labuschagne, Lock, and Le Grange (2012) have examined the role of culture in determining the levels of EE in EDs in a sample of AN patients from Chicago and found that white family caregivers expressed more Warmth and Positive Remarks toward the patients than ethnic minority families, while few differences were found in Criticism or EOI. However, in other study with BN patients, no differences in EE were found between white and minority families (Hoste & Le Grange, 2008).

Given that no more studies have been found in ED from a cultural perspective of EE, another way of approximation to the issue has been considered. The literature pertaining to the experience of family members living with or caring for an individual with an ED was recently systematically reviewed by Anastasiadou, Medina-Pradas, Sepulveda, and Treasure (2014). If these results are analyzed from a trans-cultural perspective to see how geographical origin and/or ethnicity impact on the family EE, several conclusions can be drawn (Table 8.1). First, according to the cultural characteristics of the participants of the 29 identified studies, regarding geographical origin, six studies were carried out in North America (U.S.A. and Canada), two studies in Australia, two studies in China, and 19 in Europe. Concerning the ethnic groups under study, samples of Anglo-Saxons and Scandinavians were analyzed in 19 studies, Mediterranean samples in eight studies, and Asian samples in two studies, although some of them were minorities in some of the studies.

Table 8.1 Descriptive data of patients, carers, and EE scores from the 18 studios selected by Anastasiadou et al. (2014), including new information of place of study and ethnic group of samples

Study	Patients						Carees					Scores	
Authors (year of publication)	Place (city, country)	*n*	Ethnic Group (%)	Diagnosis (%)	Age (mean, SD)	Illness Duration in Years (mean, SD)	*n*	Type of Relative (%)	Gender (%)	Living With Sufferer (%)	>21 Contact Hours per Week (%)	Measure Cut-off Point	EE Indices (mean, SD) High EE (%)
Medina-Pradas, Navarro, López, Grau, and Obiols (2011a, 2011b)	Barcelona, Spain	77	White = 100	AN = 46.7 BN = 31.2 EDNOS = 22.1	26.4 (7.3)	8.8 (6.6)	77	Mother: 70.1 Father: 5.2 Other: 24.7	F: 72.7 M: 27.3	79.2	81.8	CFI EE indices High EE High CC (≥6) High EOI (0–5/≥6)	CC: 5.0 (3.8) EOI: 1.9 (0–5) W: 3.21 (0–5) PR: 3.0 (2.4) 49.4% 33.8% 28.6%
Sepulveda, Todd, Whitaker, Grover, Stahl, and Treasure (2010)	London, UK	45	NR	AN = 77.8 BN = 22.1	21.5 (5.3)	3.07 (3.1)	47	Mother: NR Father: NR Parent: 95.7 Other: 4.3	F: 91.5 M: 8.5	76.1	62.2	FMSS High EE High CC (≥1) High EOI (≥3)	55.3% 19.1% 36.2%
Duclos et al. (2013)	Paris, France	60	NR	AN = 91.7 Other = 8.3	16.6 (1.6)	1.38 (0.6)	118	Mother: 50.8 Father: 49.2	F: 50.8 M: 49.2	100	NR	FMSS Mother high EE Mother high CC (≥1) Mother high EOI (≥3) Father high EE Father high CC (≥1) Father high EOI (≥3)	51.7% 24.1% 36.2% 49.1% 27.3% 34.5%

Grover et al. (2011b)	London, UK	27	NR	AN-R = 70.4 AN-P = 18.5 EDNOS = 7.4 Recovered = 3.7	28 (9.5)	7.1 (8.4)	27	Mother: 63 Father: 11.1 Parent: 74.1 Other: 25.9	NR	77.8	NR	FMSS High EE High CC (≥1) High EOI (≥3)	 37%
Hoste et al. (2012)	Chicago, IL, U.S.A.	189	White = 76.2 Asian = 10.1 Latino = 7.9 Other = 5.8	AN = 100	14.7 (1.6)	0.9 (0.8)	344	Mother: 53.5 Father: 46.5	F: 53.5 M: 46.5	100	NR	SCFI indices High EE High EE-CC (≥6) High EE-EOI (≥3)	Father CC = 0.4 (1.0) Mother CC = 0.5 (1.7) Father EOI = 0.4 (0.7) Mother EOI = 0.8 (1.0) Father W = 1.54 (1.3) Mother W = 2.1 (1.2) Father PR = 1.0 (1.3) Mother PR = 1.6 (1.7) White: 30.5 % Minority: 31.1 %. Mother: 2.7 % Father: 0.6 % Mother: 8.2 % Father: 1.9 %

(Continued)

Table 8.1 (Continued)

Study		Patients					Carees					Scores	
Authors (year of publication)	**Place (city, country)**	***n***	**Ethnic Group (%)**	**Diagnosis (%)**	**Age (mean, SD)**	**Illness Duration in Years (mean, SD)**	***n***	**Type of Relative (%)**	**Gender (%)**	**Living With Sufferer (%)**	**>21 Contact Hours per Week (%)**	**Measure Cut-off Point**	**EE Indices (mean, SD) High EE (%)**
Gísladóttir and Svavarsdóttir (2011)	Reykjavik, Iceland	14	NR	AN = 21.4 BN = 57.2 EDNOS= 7.1 Unknown = 14.3	21 (NR)	NR	24	Mother: 48 Father: 28 Other: 24	NR	NR	NR	LEE (0–60/≥9)	12.3 (9.5)
Grover et al. (2011a)	London, UK	63	NR	AN-R = 60.3 AN-P = 17.5 EDNOS = 20.6 Unknown = 1.6	20.4 (6.2)	4.3 (4.5)	63	Mother: 79.4 Father: 7.9 Parent: 87.3 Other: 12.7	NR	77.8	NR	LEE (0–60/≥9)	11.1 (9.6)
Grover et al. (2011b)	London, UK	27	NR	AN-R = 70.4 AN-P = 18,5 EDNOS = 7.4 Recovered = 3.7	28 (9.5)	7.1 (8.4)	27	Mother: 63 Father: 11.1 Parent: 74.1 Other: 25.9	NR	77.8	NR	LEE (0–60/≥9)	12.5 (6.6)

Sepulveda, Anastasiadou, del Rio, and Graell (2012)	Madrid, Spain	186	White = 100	AN = 68.8 BN = 31.2	20.9 (7.2)	4.2 (4.8)	270	NR	F: 63 M: 37	84.9	77.3	LEE (0–45) (0–60/≥9)	11.1 (6.1) 14.8 (8.1)
Sepulveda, Kyriacou, and Treasure (2009)	London, UK	193	NR	AN = 70.5 BN = 24.4 Unclear = 5.1	21.3 (6.8)	5.9 (5.9)	193	Mother: NR Father: NR Parent: 90.7 Other: 9.3	F: 85.5 M: 14.5	78	60.6	FQ-CC (10–40) FQ-EOI (10–40) High CC (≥23) High EOI (≥27)	23.4 (5.5) 28.2 (4.4) 56.1% 65.4%
Gísladóttir and Svavarsdóttir (2011)	Reykjavik, Iceland	14	NR	AN = 21.4 BN = 57.2 EDNOS = 7.1 Unknown = 14.3	21 (NR)	NR	24	Mother: 48 Father: 28 Other: 24	NR	NR	NR	FQ-CC (10–40) FQ-EOI (10–40) High CC (≥23) High EOI (≥27)	21.7 (4.8) 24.8 (5.0) NR NR
Goddard et al. (2011)	London, UK	142	NR	AN = 85.9 BN = 8.5 EDNOS = 5.6	20.9 (9.7)	3.5 (9.9)	153	Mother: 85 Father: 5.9 Parent: 90.9 Other: 9.2	F: 88.9 M: 11.1	76.5	58.2	FQ-CC (10–40) FQ-EOI (10–40) High CC (≥23) High EOI (≥27)	23.2 (5.6) 28.4 (4.4) 53.1% 66.7%
Coomber and King (2012)	Victoria, Australia	56	White = 100	AN = 67.9 BN = 12.5 Combination = 1.8 Unknown = 7.1 BE = 1.8	21.5 (8.7)	5.1 (5.0)	56	Mother: NR Father: NR Parent: 75 Other: 25	F: 78.6 M: 21.4	78.5	NR	FQ-CC (10–40) FQ-EOI (10–40) High CC (≥23) High EOI (≥27)	25.8 (5.8) 31.1 (3.4) 73.2% 89.3%

(Continued)

Table 8.1 (Continued)

Study		Patients					Carees					Scores	
Authors (year of publication)	**Place (city, country)**	***n***	**Ethnic Group (%)**	**Diagnosis (%)**	**Age (mean, SD)**	**Illness Duration in Years (mean, SD)**	***n***	**Type of Relative (%)**	**Gender (%)**	**Living With Sufferer (%)**	**>21 Contact Hours per Week (%)**	**Measure Cut-off Point**	**EE Indices (mean, SD) High EE (%)**
Pépin and King (2012)	Victoria, Australia	11	NR	AN = 63.6 BN = 18.2 Combination = 9.1 Unknown = 9.1	20.1 (3.0)	4.3 (3.5)	15	Mother: 73.3 Father: 26.7	F: 73.3 M: 26.7	80	NR	FQ-CC (10–40) FQ-EOI (10–40) High CC (≥23) High EOI (≥27)	24.5 (7.0) 30.5 (2.6) 64.3% 85.7%
Merwin, Zucker, and Timko (2013)	Durham, NC, U.S.A.	6	White = 83.3 African American = 16.7	AN = 100	12–18	NR	11	NR	NR	100	NR	FQ-CC (10–40) FQ-EOI (10–40) High CC (≥23) High EOI (≥27)	21.2 (6.9) 26.0 (5.5) 33.0% 44.0%
Anastasiasdou, Sepúlveda, Parks, Cuellar-Flores, and Graell (2016)	Madrid, Spain	50	White = 89.2 Latino = 10.8	AN = 78 BN = 6 EDNOS = 16	14.8 (1.8)	1.3 (1.1)	93	Mother: 51.6 Father: 48.4 Parent: 100	F: 51.6 M: 48.4	93.8	85.4	FQ-CC (10–40) FQ-EOI (10–40) High CC (≥23) High EOI (≥27)	Mother: 22.7 (5.4) Father: 20.6 (5.0) Mother: 27.1 (5.1) Father: 24.9 (4.3) Mother: 47.9% Father: 40% Mother: 58.3% Father: 28.9%

Nilsson (in preparation)	Umeå, Sweden	32	White =100	NR = 59.3	15.1 (NR)	2.0 (NR)	54	NR	NR	100	NR	FQ-CC (10–40) FQ-EOI (10–40) High CC (≥23) High EOI (≥27)	20.5 (6.0) 25.9 (5.9) NR NR
Tsiaka, Treasure, and Schmidt (in preparation)	Athens, Greece	81	NR	AN = 28.5 BN = 54.3 BED = 16 EDNOS = 1.2	25.9 (6.5)	8.8 (NR)	112	Mother: 65.2 Father: 34.8	F: 65.2 M: 34.8	63.9	NR	FQ-CC (10–40) FQ-EOI (10–40) High CC (≥23) High EOI (≥27)	21.6 (6.0) 27.3 (5.6) 36.7% 50.9%

Notes: AN = anorexia nervosa; AN-B/P = anorexia nervosa – bingeing/purging type; AN-P = anorexia nervosa – purging type; AN-R = anorexia nervosa – restrictive type; BED = binge eating disorder; BN = bulimia nervosa; CFI = Camberwell Family Interview; EDNOS = eating disorder not otherwise specified; EDNOS-B/P = eating disorder not otherwise specified – bingeing/purging type; EDNOS-R = eating disorder not otherwise specified – restrictive type; EE = expressed emotion; F = female; FMSS = Five-Minute Speech Sample; FQ-CC = Family Questionnaire – Criticism subscale; FQ-EOI = Family Questionnaire – Emotional Overinvolvement subscale; LEE = Level of Expressed Emotion scale; M = male; NR = not referred; SCFI = Standardized Clinical Family Interview.

Relatives' EE in response to ED was measured by the Family Questionnaire (FQ) (if needed, readers can go to Chapter 4 to remind themselves about assessment instruments descriptions) from a geographical view; results indicate that Criticism and EOI ratings between studies conducted in Europe (Sepulveda et al., 2009; Goddard et al., 2011; Anastasiadou et al., 2016; Svensson et al., 2013; Tsiaka, Treasure, & Schmidt, in preparation; Gísladóttir & Svavarsdóttir, 2011) and in North America (Merwin et al., 2013; Coomber & King, 2012; Pépin & King, 2012) were quite homogeneous (FQ_Criticism mean score = 22.6; FQ_EOI mean score = 25.6). Similarities among Criticism and EOI ratings were also observed when taking into account ethnic groups; for example, Anglo-Saxon or Scandinavian carers from Europe and North America (Sepulveda et al., 2009; Goddard et al., 2011; Merwin et al., 2013; Coomber & King, 2012; Pépin & King, 2012; Svensson et al., 2013; Gísladóttir & Svavarsdóttir, 2011) showed the same patterns of emotional response to the illness as Mediterranean carers (Anastasiadou et al., in preparation; Tsiaka, Treasure, & Schmidt, in preparation). Nevertheless, observing percentages of high criticism, it can be noted that Anglo-Saxon or Scandinavian ethnic groups (Sepulveda et al., 2009; Goddard et al., 2011; Merwin et al., 2013; Coomber & King, 2012; Pépin & King, 2012) had a slightly greater tendency to report high criticism than Mediterranean groups (Anastasiadou et al., 2016; Tsiaka, Treasure, & Schmidt, in preparation). The same trend was also observed among high EOI percentages, with Mediterranean carers (Anastasiadou et al., 2016; Tsiaka et al., in preparation) showing a lower propensity to get emotionally overinvolved than Anglo-Saxon or Scandinavian carers (Sepulveda et al., 2009; Goddard et al., 2011; Merwin et al., 2013; Coomber & King, 2012; Pépin & King, 2012). Nevertheless, other dimensions pertaining to ED-specific patient information, such as patient age or length of illness, or even aspects related to the perspective from which EE is measured (Medina-Pradas, 2016), as well as some demographic information that may not have been registered in some studies, must be taken into account.

The Level of Expressed Eomotion (LEE) ratings reported in four studies conducted in Europe (Grover et al., 2011a, 2011b; Gísladóttir & Svavarsdóttir, 2011; Sepúlveda et al., 2012) were also quite homogeneous among Anglo-Saxon or Scandinavian (Grover et al., 2011a, 2011b; Gísladóttir & Svavarsdóttir, 2011) and Mediterranean (Sepúlveda et al., 2012) carers (LEE mean score = 12.7). Regarding semi-structured interviews (Camberwell Family Interview [CFI] or Standardized Clinical Family Interview [SCFI]), the majority of studies were conducted in Europe (Sepulveda et al., 2010; Grover et al., 2011b; Medina-Pradas et al., 2011a, 2011b; Duclos et al., 2013), and one study was conducted in North America (Hoste et al., 2012). Results from these studies showed high criticism in 19.1% of Anglo Saxon or Scandinavians versus 33.8% among Mediterraneans, while high EOI was present in 36.2% of the Anglo-Saxon or Scandinavian samples versus 28.6% of Mediterraneans. These results indicate an inversely proportional relationship between Critical Comments and EOI.

EE ratings between different countries and cultures were therefore quite homogeneous. Anglo-Saxon or Scandinavian ED carers from Europe and North America, as well as Mediterranean carers, caring for ED patients with different characteristics (e.g., illness duration ranging from one to seven years, ages corresponding to adolescents and/or adults) responded emotionally to the illness in a similar way.

Overall, the existing literature demonstrates that, across cultures, there are no differences in the negative aspects of EE, while in AN (not in BN), there are cultural differences in the positive dimensions of EE. This seems to be contrary to findings in schizophrenia, as more positive aspects of EE were found in minorities compared with white individuals (fewer negative aspects were found in these populations as well). It is important to remember that EOI is perceived as warmth by relatives but perceived as criticism by patients.

Overall, it seems that research has focused more on intra-familial and individual aspects of the family caregiving in EDs, such as socio-demographic characteristics, coping strategies, or health status, than extra-familiar aspects. Little research has been conducted on how different cultural backgrounds may lead families to different emotional and behavioral responses to the illness. A growing number of researchers (Le Grange, Telch, & Agras, 1997; Hoste, Hewell, & Le Grange, 2007) have found that there may be fewer cultural differences and more similarities regarding ED presentation among ethnic groups than previously thought.

Therefore, the consolidation of conclusions from different studies at this respect still cannot be performed. The next step would be looking for personal or environmental factors that could explain differences or similarities between cultures regarding ED pathology and familial responses to ED.

References

Aguilera, A., López, S. R., Breitborde, N. J., Kopelowicz, A., & Zarate, R. (2010). Expressed emotion and sociocultural moderation in the course of schizophrenia. *Journal of Abnormal Psychology*, *119*(4), 875.

Al-Adawi, S., Dorvlo, A. S., Burke, D. T., Al-Bahlani, S., Martin, R. G., & Al-Ismaily, S. (2002). Presence and severity of anorexia and bulimia among male and female Omani and non-Omani adolescents. *Journal of the American Academy of Child & Adolescent Psychiatry*, *41*(9), 1124–1130.

Anastasiadou, D., Medina-Pradas, C., Sepulveda, A. R., & Treasure, J. (2014). A systematic review of family caregiving in eating disorders. *Eating Behaviors*, *15*(3), 464–477.

Anastasiasdou, D., Sepúlveda, A. R., Parks, M., Cuellar-Flores, I., & Graell, M. (2016). The relationship between dysfunctional family patterns and symptom severity among adolescent patients with eating disorders: A gender-specific approach. *Women & Health*, *56*(6), 695–712.

Anderson-Fye, E. P. (2004). A "Coca-Cola" shape: Cultural change, body image, and eating disorders in San Andres, Belize. *Culture, Medicine and Psychiatry*, *28*(4), 561–595.

Becker, A. E. (2007). Culture and eating disorders classification. *International Journal of Eating Disorders*, *40*(S3), S111–S116.

Becker, A. E., Burwell, R. A., Herzog, D. B., Hamburg, P., & Gilman, S. E. (2002). Eating behaviours and attitudes following prolonged exposure to television among ethnic Fijian adolescent girls. *The British Journal of Psychiatry*, *180*(6), 509–514.

Becker, A. E., Eddy, K. T., & Perloe, A. (2009). Clarifying criteria for cognitive signs and symptoms for eating disorders in DSM-V. *International Journal of Eating Disorders*, *42*(7), 611–619.

Becker, A. E., Franko, D. L., Speck, A., & Herzog, D. B. (2003). Ethnicity and differential access to care for eatingdisorder symptoms. *International Journal of Eating Disorders*, *33*, 205–212.

Bertrando, P., Beltz, J., Bressi, C., Clerici, M., Farma, T., Invernizzi, G., & Cazzullo, C. L. (1992). Expressed emotion and schizophrenia in Italy: A study of an urban population. *The British Journal of Psychiatry*, *161*(2), 223–229.

Bhugra, D., Bhui, K., & Gupta, K. R. (2000). Bulimic disorders and sociocentric values in north India. *Social Psychiatry and Psychiatric Epidemiology*, *35*(2), 86–93.

Bhugra, D., Mastrogianni, A., Maharajh, H., & Harvey, S. (2003). Prevalence of bulimic behaviours and eating attitudes in schoolgirls from Trinidad and Barbados. *Transcultural Psychiatry*, *40*(3), 409–428.

Bhugra, D., & McKenzie, K. (2003). Expressed emotion across cultures. *Advances in Psychiatric Treatment*, *9*, 342–348.

Birch, L. L., & Fisher, J. O. (1998). Development of eating behaviors among children and adolescents. *Pediatrics*, *101*, 539–549.

Brown, G. W. (1985). The discovery of expressed emotion: Induction or deduction. *Expressed Emotion in Families*, 7–25.

Cha, J. (1994). Aspects of individualism and collectivism in Korea. In U. Kim, H. C. Triandis, C. Kagitcibasi, S. Choi, & G. Yoon (Eds.), *Individualism and collectivism, theory, method, and Appllcations* (pp. 157–174). Thousand Oaks, CA: Sage Publications.

Cheng, A. T. (2002). Expressed emotion: A cross-culturally valid concept? *The British Journal of Psychiatry*, *181*(6), 466–467.

Connell, C. M., & Gibson, G. D. (1997). Racial, ethnic, and cultural differences in dementia caregiving: Review and analysis. *The Gerontologist*, *37*(3), 355–364.

Coomber, K., & King, R. M. (2012). Coping strategies and social support as predictors and mediators of eating disorder carer burden and psychological distress. *Social Psychiatry and Psychiatric Epidemiology*, *47*(5), 789–796.

Domínguez-Martínez, T., Medina-Pradas, C., Kwapil, T. R., & Barrantes-Vidal, N. (2014). Relatives' illness attributions mediate the association of expressed emotion with early psychosis symptoms and functioning. *Psychiatry Research*, *15*, *218*(1–2), 48–53.

Domínguez-Martínez, T., Medina-Pradas, C., Kwapil, T. R., & Barrantes-Vidal, N. (2017). Relatives' expressed emotion, distress and attributions in clinical high-risk and recent onset of psychosis. *Psychiatry Research*, *247*, 323–329.

Duclos, J., Maria, A. S., Dorard, G., Curt, F., Apfel, A., Vibert, S., . . . Godart, N. (2013). Bonding and expressed emotion: Two interlinked concepts? *Psychopathology*, *46*(6), 404–412.

Duclos, J., Vibert, S., Mattar, L., & Godart, N. (2012). Expressed emotion in families of patients with eating disorders: A review of the literature. *Current Psychiatry Reviews*, *8*(3), 183–202.

Eddy, K. T., Hennessey, M., & Thompson-Brenner, H. (2007). Eating pathology in East African women: The role of media exposure and globalization. *The Journal of Nervous and Mental Disease*, *195*(3), 196–202.

Fox, J. R., Dean, M., & Whittlesea, A. (2017). The experience of caring for or living with an individual with an eating disorder: A meta-synthesis of qualitative studies. *Clinical Psychology & Psychotherapy*, *24*(1), 103–125.

Franko, D. L., Becker, A. E., Thomas, J. J., & Herzog, D. B. (2007). Cross-ethnic differences in eating disorder symptoms and related distress. *International Journal of Eating Disorders*, *40*(2), 156–164.

Gilbert, S. C. (2003). Eating disorders in women of color. *Clinical Psychology: Science and Practice*, *10*(4), 444–455.

Gísladóttir, M., & Svavarsdóttir, E. K. (2011). Educational and support intervention to help families assist in the recovery of relatives with eating disorders. *Journal of Psychiatric and Mental Health Nursing*, *18*(2), 122–130.

Goddard, E., Macdonald, P., Sepulveda, A. R., Naumann, U., Landau, S., Schmidt, U., & Treasure, J. (2011). Cognitive interpersonal maintenance model of eating disorders: Intervention for carers. *The British Journal of Psychiatry*, *199*(3), 225–231.

Gordon, K. H., Perez, M., & Joiner, T. E., Jr. (2002). The impact of racial stereotypes on eating disorder recognition. *International Journal of Eating Disorders*, *32*(2), 219–224.

Grover, M., Naumann, U., Mohammad-Dar, L., Glennon, D., Ringwood, S., Eisler, I., . . . Schmidt, U. (2011a). A randomized controlled trial of an Internet-based cognitive-behavioural skills package for carers of people with anorexia nervosa. *Psychological Medicine*, *41*(12), 2581–2591.

Grover, M., Williams, C., Eisler, I., Fairbairn, P., McCloskey, C., Smith, G., . . . Schmidt, U. (2011b). An off-line pilot evaluation of a web-based systemic cognitive-behavioral intervention for carers of people with anorexia nervosa. *International Journal of Eating Disorders*, *44*(8), 708–715.

Gutiérrez, E., Sepúlveda, A. R., Anastasiadou, D., & Medina-Pradas, C. (2014). Programa de Psicoeducación Familiar para Trastornos del Comportamiento Alimentario. *Behavioral Psychology/Psicologia Conductual*, *22*(1), 133–152.

Hall, G. C. N. (2001). Psychotherapy research with ethnic minorities: Empirical, ethical, and conceptual issues. *Journal of Consulting and Clinical Psychology*, *69*(3), 502.

Haworth-Hoeppner, S. (2000). The critical shape of body image: The role of culture and the family in the production of eating disorders. *Journal of Marriage and the Family, 62*, 212–227.
Heresco-Levy, U., Greenberg, D., & Dasberg, H. (1990). Family expressed emotion: Concepts, dilemmas and the Israeli perspective. *Israel Journal of Psychiatry and Related Sciences, 27*(4), 205–215.
Hoek, H. W. (2006). Incidence, prevalence and mortality of anorexia nervosa and other eating disorders. *Current Opinion in Psychiatry, 19*(4), 389–394.
Hoek, H. W., van Harten, P. N., Hermans, K. M., Katzman, M. A., Matroos, G. E., & Susser, E. S. (2005). The incidence of anorexia nervosa on Curacao. *American Journal of Psychiatry, 162*(4), 748–752.
Hoste, R. R., Hewell, K., & Le Grange, D. (2007). Family interaction among white and ethnic minority adolescents with bulimia nervosa and their parents. *European Eating Disorders Review: The Professional Journal of the Eating Disorders Association, 15*(2), 152–158.
Hoste, R. R., Labuschagne, Z., Lock, J., & Le Grange, D. (2012). Cultural variability in expressed emotion among families of adolescents with anorexia nervosa. *International Journal of Eating Disorders, 45*(1), 142–145.
Hoste, R. R., & Le Grange, D. (2008). Expressed emotion among white and ethnic minority families of adolescents with bulimia nervosa. *European Eating Disorders Review: The Professional Journal of the Eating Disorders Association, 16*(5), 395–400.
Jenkins, J. H. (1991). The 1990 Stirling Award essay: Anthropology, expressed emotion, and schizophrenia. *Ethos, 19*, 387–431.
Jenkins, J. H., & Karno, M. (1992). The meaning of expressed emotion: Theoretical issues raised by cross-cultural research. *American Journal of Psychiatry, 149*, 9–21.
Jenkins, J. H., Karno, M., de la Selva, A., & Santana, F. (1986). Expressed emotion in cross-cultural context: Familial responses to schizophrenic illness among Mexican Americans. In *Treatment of schizophrenia* (pp. 35–49). Berlin, Heidelberg: Springer-Verlag.
Kamal, A. (1995). Variables in expressed emotion associated with relapse: A comparison between depressed and schizophrenic samples in an Egyptian community. *Current Psychiatry, 2*(2), 211–216.
Kaplan, R. (1966). Cultural thought patterns in inter-cultural education. *Language Learning, 16*, 1–20.
Katzman, M. A., Hermans, K. M., Van Hoeken, D., & Hoek, H. W. (2004). Not your "typical island woman": Anorexia nervosa is reported only in subcultures in Curacao. *Culture, Medicine and Psychiatry, 28*(4), 463–492.
Kavanagh, D. J. (1992). Recent developments in expressed emotion and schizophrenia. *British Journal of Psychiatry, 160*, 601–620.
Keel, P. K., & Klump, K. L. (2003). Are eating disorders culture-bound syndromes? Implications for conceptualizing their etiology. *Psychological Bulletin, 129*(5), 747.
Kopelowicz, A., Zarate, R., Gonzalez, V., López, S. R., Ortega, P., Obregon, N., & Mintz, J. (2002). Evaluation of expressed emotion in schizophrenia: A comparison of Caucasians and Mexican-Americans. *Schizophrenia Research, 55*(1–2), 179–186.
Kuipers, L. (1987). Research in expressed emotion. *Social Psychiatry and Psychiatric Epidemiology, 22*(4), 216–220.
Kymalainen, J. A., & Weisman de Mamani, A. G. (2008). Expressed emotion, communication deviance, and culture in families of patients with schizophrenia: A review of the literature. *Cultural Diversity & Ethnic Minority Psychology, 14*, 85–91.
Kymalainen, J. A., Weisman, A. G., Rosales, G. A., & Armesto, J. C. (2006). Ethnicity, expressed emotion, and communication deviance in family members of patients with schizophrenia. *The Journal of Nervous and Mental Disease, 194*(6), 391–396.

Lee, S., Kwok, K., Liau, C., & Leung, T. (2002). Screening Chinese patients with eating disorders using the Eating Attitudes Test in Hong Kong. *International Journal of Eating Disorders, 32*, 91–97.

Lee, S., Lee, A. M., Ngai, E., Lee, D. T., & Wing, Y. K. (2001). Rationales for food refusal in Chinese patients with anorexia nervosa. *International Journal of Eating Disorders, 29*(2), 224–229.

Lee, S., Ng, K. L., Kwok, K., & Fung, C. (2010). The changing profile of eating disorders at a tertiary psychiatric clinic in Hong Kong (1987–2007). *International Journal of Eating Disorders, 43*(4), 307–314.

Leff, J., & Vaughn, C. (1985). *Expressed emotion in families: Its significance for mental illness.* New York: Guilford Press.

Lefley, H. P. (1987). Culture and mental illness: The family role. In A. B. Hatfield & H. P. Lefley (Eds.), *Families of mentally ill: Coping and adaptation.* New York: Guilford Press.

Le Grange, D., Telch, C. F., & Agras, W. S. (1997). Eating and general psychopathology in a sample of Caucasian and ethnic minority subjects. *International Journal of Eating Disorders, 21*(3), 285–293.

López, S. R., Ramírez García, J. I., Ullman, J. B., Kopelowicz, A., Jenkins, J., Breitborde, N. J., & Placencia, P. (2009). Cultural variability in the manifestation of expressed emotion. *Family Process, 48*(2), 179–194.

Makino, M., Tsuboi, K., & Dennerstein, L. (2004). Prevalence of eating disorders: A comparison of Western and non-Western countries. *MedGenMed: Medscape General Medicine, 6*(3), 49.

Markey, C. N. (2004). Culture and the development of eating disorders: A tripartite model. *Eating Disorders, 12*(2), 139–156.

Medina-Pradas, C. (2016). Actualización en torno a la Emoción Expresada: Consideraciones teóricas, metodológicas y prácticas. *Revista de Psicoterapia, 27*(103), 251–266.

Medina-Pradas, C., Navarro, J. B., López, S. R., Grau, A., & Obiols, J. E. (2011a). Further development of a scale of perceived expressed emotion and its evaluation in a sample of patients with eating disorders. *Psychiatry Research, 190*(2–3), 291–296.

Medina-Pradas, C., Navarro, J. B., López, S. R., Grau, A., & Obiols, J. E. (2011b). Dyadic view of expressed emotion, stress, and eating disorder psychopathology. *Appetite, 57*(3), 743–748.

Medina-Pradas, C., Navarro, J. B., Pousa, E., Montero, M. I., & Obiols, J. E. (2013). Expressed and perceived criticism, family warmth, and symptoms in schizophrenia. *Spanish Journal of Psychology, 16*, e45, 1–8.

Meneghelli, A., Alpi, A., Pafumi, N., Patelli, G., Preti, A., & Cocchi, A. (2011). Expressed emotion in first-episode schizophrenia and in ultra high-risk patients: Results from the Programma 2000 (Milan, Italy). *Psychiatry Research, 189*(3), 331–338.

Merwin, R. M., Zucker, N. L., & Timko, C. A. (2013). A pilot study of an acceptance-based separated family treatment for adolescent anorexia nervosa. *Cognitive and Behavioral Practice, 20*(4), 485–500.

Miller, M. N., & Pumariega, A. J. (2001). Culture and eating disorders: A historical and cross-cultural review. *Psychiatry, 64*(2), 93–110.

Mottaghipour, Y., Pourmand, D., Maleki, H., & Davidian, L. (2001). Expressed emotion and the course of schizophrenia in Iran. *Social Psychiatry and Psychiatric Epidemiology, 36*(4), 195–199.

Nasser, M. (2009). Eating disorders across cultures. *Psychiatry, 8*(9), 347–350.

Nasser, M., & Katzman, M. (1999). Eating disorders: Transcultural perspectives inform prevention. *Preventing Eating Disorders: A Handbook of Interventions and Special Challenges*, 26–43.

Njenga, F. G., & Kangethe, R. N. (2004). Anorexia nervosa in Kenya. *East African Medical Journal, 81*, 188–193.

Nomura, H., Inoue, S., Kamimura, N., Shimodera, S., Mino, Y., Gregg, L., & Tarrier, N. (2005). A cross-cultural study on expressed emotion in carers of people with dementia and schizophrenia: Japan and England. *Social Psychiatry and Psychiatric Epidemiology*, *40*(7), 564–570.

Okasha, A., El Akabawi, A. S., Snyder, K. S., Wilson, A. K., Youssef, I., & El Dawla, A. S. (1994). Expressed emotion, perceived criticism, and relapse in depression: A replication in an Egyptian community. *American Journal of Psychiatry*, *151*, 1001–1005.

Pavlova, B., Uher, R., Dragomirecka, E., & Papezova, H. (2010). Trends in hospital admissions for eating disorders in a country undergoing a socio-cultural transition, the Czech Republic 1981–2005. *Social Psychiatry and Psychiatric Epidemiology*, *45*(5), 541–550.

Pavlova, B., Uher, R., & Papezova, H. (2008). It would not have happened to me at home: Qualitative exploration of sojourns abroad and eating disorders in young Czech women. *European Eating Disorders Review: The Professional Journal of the Eating Disorders Association*, *16*(3), 207–214.

Pépin, G., & King, R. (2012). Collaborative care skills training workshops: Helping carers cope with eating disorders from the UK to Australia. *Social Psychiatry and Psychiatric Epidemiology*, *48*(5), 805–812.

Phillips, M. R., & Xiong, W. (1995). Expressed emotion in mainland China: Chinese families with schizophrenic patients. *International Journal of Mental Health*, *24*, 54–75.

Pike, K. M., Dohm, F. A., Striegel-Moore, R. H., Wilfley, D. E., & Fairburn, C. G. (2001). A comparison of black and white women with binge eating disorder. *American Journal of Psychiatry*, *158*(9), 1455–1460.

Podar, I., & Allik, J. (2009). A cross-cultural comparison of the Eating Disorder Inventory. *International Journal of Eating Disorders*, *42*(4), 346–355.

Pumariega, A. J., & Cross, T. L. (1997). Cultural competence in child psychiatry. *Basic Handbook of Child and Adolescent Psychiatry*, *4*, 473–484.

Ramírez García, J. I., Wood, J. M., Hosch, H. M., & Meyer, L. M. (2004). Predicting psychiatric rehospitalizations: The role of Latino versus European American ethnicity. *Psychological Services*, *1*, 147–157.

Scherer, K. R., Clark-Polner, E., & Mortillaro, M. (2011). In the eye of the beholder? Universality and cultural specificity in the expression and perception of emotion. *International Journal of Psychology*, *46*(6), 401–435.

Sepúlveda, A. R., Anastasiadou, D., del Río, A. M., & Graell, M. (2012). The Spanish validation of level of expressed emotion scale for relatives of people with eating disorders. *The Spanish Journal of Psychology*, *15*(2), 825–839.

Sepulveda, A. R., Kyriacou, O., & Treasure, J. (2009). Development and validation of the Accommodation and Enabling Scale for Eating Disorders (AESED) for caregivers in eating disorders. *BMC Health Services Research*, *9*(1), 171.

Sepulveda, A. R., Todd, G., Whitaker, W., Grover, M., Stahl, D., & Treasure, J. (2010). Expressed emotion in relatives of patients with eating disorders following skills training program. *International Journal of Eating Disorders*, *43*(7), 603–610.

Shweder, R. A., & LeVine, R. A. (1984). *Culture theory: Essays on mind, self, and emotion*. Cambridge: Cambridge University Press.

Siefert, M. L., Williams, A. L., Dowd, M. F., Chappel-Aiken, L., & McCorkle, R. (2008). The caregiving experience in a racially diverse sample of cancer family caregivers. *Cancer Nursing*, *31*(5), 399.

Singelis, T. M. (1994). The measurement of independent and interdependent selfconstruals. *Personality and Social Psychology Bulletin*, *20*, 580–591.

Singh, S. P., Harley, K., & Suhail, K. (2013). Cultural specificity of emotional overinvolvement: A systematic review. *Schizophrenia Bulletin*, *39*(2), 449–463.

Snowden, L. R. (2007). Explaining mental health treatment disparities: Ethnic and cultural differences in family involvement. *Culture, Medicine and Psychiatry*, *31*(3), 389–402.
Soh, N. L. W., Touyz, S. W., & Surgenor, L. J. (2006). Eating and body image disturbances across cultures: A review. *European Eating Disorders Review: The Professional Journal of the Eating Disorders Association*, *14*(1), 54–65.
Soh, N. L. W., & Walter, G. (2013). Publications on cross-cultural aspects of eating disorders. *Journal of Eating Disorders*, *1*(1), 4.
Striegel-Moore, R. H., Dohm, F. A., Kraemer, H. C., Taylor, C. B., Daniels, S., Crawford, P. B., & Schreiber, G. B. (2003). Eating disorders in white and black women. *American Journal of Psychiatry*, *160*(7), 1326–1331.
Svensson, E., Nilsson, K., Levi, R., & Suarez, N. C. (2013). *Parents' experiences of having and caring for a child with an eating disorder. Eating disorders*, *21*(5), 395–407.
Thomas, C. L., James, A. C., & Bachmann, M. O. (2002). Eating attitudes in English secondary school students: Influences of ethnicity, gender, mood, and social class. *International Journal of Eating Disorders*, *31*(1), 92–96.
Thomas, J. J., Crosby, R. D., Wonderlich, S. A., Striegel-Moore, R. H., & Becker, A. E. (2011). A latent profile analysis of the typology of bulimic symptoms in an indigenous Pacific population: Evidence of cross-cultural variation in phenomenology. *Psychological Medicine*, *41*(1), 195–206.
Treasure, J., & Nazar, B. P. (2016). Interventions for the carers of patients with eating disorders. *Current Psychiatry Reports*, *18*(2), 16.
Treasure, J., & Schmidt, U. (2013). The cognitive-interpersonal maintenance model of anorexia nervosa revisited: A summary of the evidence for cognitive, socio-emotional and interpersonal predisposing and perpetuating factors. *Journal of Eating Disorders*, *15*, 1–13.
Tsai, G. (2000). Eating disorders in the Far East. *Eating and Weight Disorders-Studies on Anorexia, Bulimia and Obesity*, *5*(4), 183–197.
Tsiaka, M., Treasure, J., & Schmidt, U. Eating disorders in Greece: Examination of parents' distress, attitudes and behaviors (Submitted).
Vaughn, C. E. (1989). Expressed emotion in family relationships. *Child Psychology & Psychiatry & Allied Disciplines*, *30*(1), 13–22.
Wearden, A. J., Tarrier, N., & Barrowclough, C., (2000). A review of expressed emotion research in health care. *Clinical Psychology Review*, *20*, 633–666.
Weisman, A. G. (2005). Integrating culturally-based approaches with existing interventions for Hispanic/Latino families coping with schizophrenia. *Psychotherapy: Theory, Research, Practice, Training*, *42*, 178–197.
Weisman, A. G., López, S. R., Karno, M., & Jenkins, J. (1993). An attributional analysis of expressed emotion in Mexican-American families with schizophrenia. *Journal of Abnormal Psychology*, *102*(4), 601.
Weisman de Mamani, A. G. W., Kymalainen, J. A., Rosales, G. A., & Armesto, J. C. (2007). Expressed emotion and interdependence in White and Latino/Hispanic family members of patients with schizophrenia. *Psychiatry Research*, *151*(1–2), 107–113.
Wildes, J. E., Emery, R. E., & Simons, A. D. (2001). The roles of ethnicity and culture in the development of eating disturbance and body dissatisfaction: A meta-analytic review. *Clinical Psychology Review*, *21*(4), 521–551.
Winkleby, M. A., Gardener, C. D., & Taylor, C. B. (1996). The influence of gender and socioeconomic factors on Hispanic/White differences in body mass index. *Preventative Medicine*, *25*, 203–211.

9

Factors Associated With High Expressed Emotion Versus Low Expressed Emotion

Kathryn M. Huryk and Eric F. van Furth

Despite more than five decades of longitudinal research linking caregivers' level of expressed emotion (EE) to mental health outcomes (Brown, Birley, & Wing, 1972), the mechanism of action underlying this relationship remains elusive across domains of psychopathology (Peris & Miklowitz, 2015). Understanding the factors associated with varying levels of EE can enable researchers and clinicians to pursue potentially modifiable targets for intervention. The broader concept of EE captures both positive aspects of caregivers' communication to the ill individual, such as expressions of Warmth (W) and Positive Remarks (PR), in addition to negative features, which include Emotional Overinvolvement (EOI), Critical Comments (CC), and Hostility (H) (Brown et al., 1972). When these negative features predominate a caregivers' attitude towards the ill individual, they are said to have high levels of EE. Alternatively, caregivers who demonstrate a lower frequency of these negative attitudes are considered to have low levels of EE. Within the field of eating disorders (EDs), there has been a marked emphasis on examining the correlates of negative caregiver presentations, given early evidence that high EE is associated with negative outcomes in treatment and recovery (Le Grange, Eisler, Dare, & Hodes, 1992; Le Grange, Eisler, Dare, & Russell, 1992; Szmukler, Eisler, Russell, & Dare, 1985). This focus on high EE is reflected in the literature reviewed here, which addresses the patient, parent, and family factors that are associated with level of EE amongst caregivers.

It is important to keep in mind that parents and other carers of those with EDs do not uniformly present with high EE, nor can it be assumed that their attitudes at the time of assessment are consistent with their pre-illness presentation. There is considerable evidence to suggest that these individuals may be more likely to have moderate to high levels of EE, particularly in the domains of EOI and CC (Coomber & King, 2012, 2013; Di Paola, Faravelli, & Ricca, 2010; Goddard, Hibbs, et al., 2013; Goddard, Salerno, et al., 2013; Kyriacou, Treasure, & Schmidt, 2008; Zabala, Macdonald, & Treasure, 2009). However, there is also a great deal of data indicating that parents of individuals with ED demonstrate low EE (Blondin, Meilleur, Taddeo, & Frappier, 2019; Duclos et al., 2013, 2014; Le Grange, Eisler, Dare, & Hodes, 1992; Le Grange, Hoste, Lock, & Bryson, 2011; Rienecke, Accurso, Lock, & Le Grange, 2016; Rienecke, Lebow, Lock, & Le Grange, 2017; Hoste, Labuschagne, Lock, & Le Grange, 2012; van Furth et al., 1996). Norms drawn from prior community and healthy comparator research have typically served as the standards of comparison in these studies, although there are some exceptions in which control or other illness-affected groups were used for direct comparison. The literature on EE and its relationship to ED are muddled by variations in both the method of EE measurement (see Chapter 4) and sampling, as these findings were drawn from populations that varied in age, diagnosis, illness severity, and type of caregiver. Indeed, each of these factors has been associated with differences in level of caregiver EE, as will be reviewed. Most studies of EE in ED have drawn their samples from treatment studies or higher level of care settings (e.g., inpatient and partial hospitalization programs), such that this literature may represent a subsection of families experiencing ED. Furthermore, an overwhelming majority of these studies employed cross-sectional designs, and theories describing causal relationships between EE and ED could only be substantiated with rigorous longitudinal examination or experimental manipulation.

Patient Factors Associated With Level of EE

The first avenue of research into factors associated with parental EE is illness-related factors such as symptom severity, the duration of illness, and diagnosis. More recently, the patients' EE attitude has also been investigated.

Symptom Severity

The relationships between caregiver EE and patient level variables in ED, including symptom severity and duration of illness, have been transdiagnostically replicated with few exceptions. Higher ED severity tends to be associated with higher levels of EE amongst caregivers (Goddard, Salerno, et al., 2013; Kyriacou et al., 2008; Rienecke et al., 2017; Schwarte et al., 2017). In transdiagnostic adolescent ED groups, high maternal CC has been positively correlated with ED psychopathology (Rienecke & Richmond, 2017). For anorexia nervosa (AN) specifically, high EE amongst parents has been associated with lower weight status at baseline (Eisler et al., 2000; Eisler, Simic, Russell, & Dare, 2007), although some studies suggest that AN severity may be more closely related to either maternal CC (Duclos et al., 2014) or EOI (Blair, Freeman, & Cull, 1995; Duclos, Vibert, Mattar, & Godart, 2012). This relationship between higher levels of AN severity and higher levels of EE has sometimes failed to be replicated (Le Grange et al., 2011; Rienecke, Accurso, et al., 2016; Allan, Le Grange, Sawyer, McLean, & Hughes, 2018; Hoste et al., 2012). In a study of bulimia nervosa (BN) alone, EE was not related to ED psychopathology (Hoste & Le Grange, 2008). However, others have shown that there is a relationship between high EE and greater levels of negative affect and depression in BN (Hedlund, Fichter, Quadflieg, & Brandl, 2003). Likewise, there appears to be some relationship between high EE and greater depressive symptoms amongst individuals with AN (Schwarte et al., 2017).

At the time of this writing, three studies had explicitly focused on patients' perceptions of their carers' EE, as assessed through subjective questionnaires rather than objective interview-based assessments. Of these, two evinced a positive correlation between EE and ED symptomatology in transdiagnostic samples of adult women (Di Paola et al., 2010; Medina-Pradas, Blas Navarro, López, Grau, & Obiols, 2011). The third, a pilot study that drew results from a small sample ($N = 17$) consisting of adolescent and young adult women with AN only, did not find evidence to support a relationship between EE and ED symptomatology (Moulds et al., 2000). Patients' perceptions of high EE amongst their caregivers have been associated with increased feelings of stress (Medina-Pradas et al., 2011) and guilt (Di Paola et al., 2010). Alternatively, patients' perceptions of carers' warmth were negatively related to symptom severity and stress (Medina-Pradas et al., 2011).

Medina-Pradas and colleagues (2011) furthermore demonstrated a lack of concordance between patients' perceptions of caregiver EE and the styles of communication those caregivers actually demonstrated on interview measures of EE. In this study, interview methods of assessment did not support a significant relationship between EE and ED symptomatology or stress. The authors speculate that in the act of appraising their caregivers' EE, individuals introduce additional variables that could account for the discrepancy between their subjective experience and more objective data. For example, studies of women in community settings have shown that those with elevated concerns about eating, shape, and weight hold beliefs that displaying emotion is a potentially harmful act of weakness that should be controlled (Meyer, Leung, Barry, & De Feo, 2010). If patients with ED hold such attitudes toward emotion, this could influence their experience of carers' EE and heighten their sensitivity to the negative aspects of EE. Likewise, temperamental traits associated with ED may influence the individuals' perception of carers' EE. Individuals with AN tend to be more emotionally inhibited, harm avoidant, and sensitive to negative emotionality (Kaye, Fudge, & Paulus, 2009; Klump et al., 2000), which could amplify their experience of parental criticism. Beyond the field of ED, researchers have hypothesized that heightened stress reactivity may serve as a mechanistic link between parental EE and a more deleterious course of illness (Peris & Miklowitz, 2015). Initial evidence supports a relationship between high parental EE and biomarkers of elevated stress reactivity (Christiansen, Oades, Psychogiou, Hauffa, & Sonuga-Barke, 2010; Hibbs, Zahn, Hamburger, Kruesi, & Rapoport, 1992) as well as distinct patterns of neural response (Hooley et al., 2009; Hooley, Gruber, Scott, Hiller, & Yurgelun-Todd, 2005) in offspring with psychopathology.

Duration of Illness

Elevated EE, particularly high levels of CC, has been associated with longer duration of ED illness and more advanced age of the patient

(Allan et al., 2018; Anastasiadou, Medina-Pradas, Sepulveda, & Treasure, 2014; Duclos et al., 2012, 2014; Eisler et al., 2007; Hoste et al., 2012; Szmukler et al., 1985; Zabala et al., 2009). At least two studies failed to find a relationship between duration of illness and EE, but this includes a study of patients with recent onset (Schwarte et al., 2017) and a study of adults that employed subjective perceptions of caregivers' EE (Di Paola et al., 2010). Although one can only speculate as to why high EE is associated with longer duration of illness, it is plausible that the relationship is bidirectional. When parents are confronted with the behavioral manifestations of an ED and the cumulative functional consequences of the disease over longer periods of time, they may become increasingly frustrated and feel increasingly powerless and thus vulnerable to making Critical Comments or becoming emotionally overinvolved. Relatedly, greater numbers of treatment episodes have been linked to higher levels of parental criticism (Santonastaso, Saccon, & Favaro, 1997). This suggests that when the illness does not remit despite repeated attempts at intervention, carers may be more likely to misattribute the illness's persistence to the volition of their child. However, data from the intervention literature suggests a complicated interplay between caregiver EE and treatment outcomes (Allan et al., 2018; Eisler et al., 2000; Le Grange et al., 1992; Rienecke et al., 2016), which could hypothetically contribute to longer duration of illness.

Diagnosis

The relationship between specific ED features or diagnoses and level of carer EE is not entirely clear. Some studies have shown that parents of patients with BN demonstrate higher levels of CC than those of patients with AN (Duclos et al., 2012; Rienecke, Sim, Lock, & Le Grange, 2016; van Furth et al., 1996). When caregiver EE was assessed via patient report in an adult sample, this relationship was not shown (Di Paola et al., 2010). Greater discussion of EE in AN and BN can be found elsewhere in this text (see Chapters 5 and 6, respectively).

There is a relative dearth of research on EE amongst caregivers of individuals with binge-eating disorder (BED). One study compared levels of EE between the parents of patients with BED and healthy control participants (Schmidt, Tetzlaff, & Hilbert, 2015). Patients with BED perceived their parents to have higher levels of EE, particularly higher CC, compared with the healthy control group. In this study, higher levels of perceived EE also explained a significant proportion of the variance in global ED psychopathology (Schmidt et al., 2015). Likewise, there is a lack of research examining the way in which parental EE relates to specific eating behaviors. Munsch and colleagues (2017) demonstrated that higher parental CC and EOI were correlated with higher rates of emotional eating amongst their children. Furthermore, this relationship was mediated by the children's negative urgency, or tendency to impulsively engage in behaviors during intensive mood states (Munsch et al., 2017). Additional research regarding parental attitudes and communication as pertain to specific eating behaviors is warranted.

Patient EE

Although there are evident links between caregivers' EE and patients' ED-related behaviors, the direction of causality remains unclear. EE researchers have typically been concerned with evaluating the parent's EE attitude toward the patient without, in turn, assessing the patient's EE attitude toward their parent. Two recent studies have tested the relationship between parent and child EE in adolescents with ED who were presenting for family-based treatment (Hoste, Lebow, & Le Grange, 2015; Rienecke, Lebow, et al., 2017). The first concerned adolescents with BN and demonstrated positive correlations between adolescents and their parents on CC, PR, and W (Hoste et al., 2015). To examine whether the family's overall EE profile and "fit" between parent and child EE related to treatment outcomes, patients were grouped into four categories: low patient/low parent EE, low patient/high parent EE, high patient/low parent EE, and high patient/high parent EE. Results suggested that the patients who shared a low-EE profile with their parents demonstrated the greatest reduction in purging behaviors. Furthermore, patients whose EE profile matched that of their parents experienced a significantly greater reduction in purging than those of the unmatched families. Patients with high EE whose parents had low EE experienced the smallest reduction in purging over the course of treatment (Hoste et al., 2015). These results seem to suggest that there is a bidirectional relationship between patients' and parents' level of EE and that EE "fit" between child and caregiver is also important.

When similar methodology was applied to a sample of patients with AN, the positive correlations between adolescents and their parents on CC, PR, and W were replicated (Rienecke, Lebow, et al., 2017). While parents' high EE was associated with higher ED psychopathology at the end of treatment, the patient's own EE status was not related to their treatment outcomes. Patients whose parents had low EE demonstrated better treatment outcomes than those with high EE, irrespective of the patient's own level of EE. Furthermore, neither "fit" nor EE family profile was related to treatment outcome. Given that adolescents with AN may express resistance to nourishment by making hostile or critical remarks toward caregivers, these findings are encouraging in their suggestion that such forms of resistance do not hinder treatment outcomes. Additional investigation of patients' EE as relates to their parents' EE and treatment outcomes could provide fruitful avenues for future research and intervention.

Caregiver Factors Associated With Level of EE

The second avenue of research looks at parent characteristics such as perceived burden of care, levels of psychological distress, coping mechanisms, and attributional style. Differences between parents and family factors will also be addressed.

Caregiver Burden

The experience of caring for someone with an ED is often challenging, thus parents often experience high levels of carer burden when their child is ill with this serious disease (Rhind et al., 2016). Carer burden includes both objective (e.g., time spent in caregiving tasks, financial strain) as well as subjective (e.g., caregiver distress) features. Cross-sectional studies have shown that high EE is associated with elevated levels of carer burden (Coomber & King, 2012; Winn et al., 2007). A longitudinal study demonstrated that high EE predicted carer burden over time (Coomber & King, 2013). Studies have shown that when the ill individual displays more difficult behaviors (e.g., disruptive or negative behavior, rejection of help), their caregiver tends to experience higher levels of EE, particularly CC (Blondin et al., 2019; Kyriacou et al., 2008). When difficult behaviors are paired with greater contact hours between the patient and their parent, the parents are more likely to report negative experiences of caregiving (Winn et al., 2007).

Additionally, there is a relationship between increased negative experiences of caregiving and high EE in parents of children with AN and BN (Blondin et al., 2019; Coomber & King, 2013; Duclos et al., 2012, 2013; Kyriacou et al., 2008; Sepulveda et al., 2010). This relationship appears to be bidirectional (Coomber & King, 2013) and may not be consistent across mothers and fathers (Blondin et al., 2019). Specifically, parents who experienced a greater sense of loss and their child's need for dependency tended to have higher levels of EE and EOI, while parents who were more frequently dealing with difficult behaviors had elevated CC (Blondin et al., 2019; Sepuvleda et al., 2010). Additionally, greater experience with positive aspects of caregiving was associated with elevated EOI but not CC (Blondin et al., 2019). It is worth noting that level of EE does not appear to be related to the level of parent–child bonding (Duclos et al., 2013).

Psychological Distress

Parents of children with ED tend to experience elevated levels of distress, including symptoms of depression and anxiety, which have positive correlations with high EE (Coomber & King, 2012, 2013; Duclos et al., 2012, 2014; Goddard, Salerno, et al., 2013; Kyriacou et al., 2008; Rienecke & Richmond, 2017; Schwarte et al., 2017; Whitney et al., 2005; Zabala et al., 2009). This relationship between high EE and elevated parental psychopathology has been replicated in other patient populations (Boger, Tompson, Briggs-Gowan, Pavlis, & Carter, 2008; Hibbs et al., 1991; McCarty & Weisz, 2002; Nelson, Hammen, Brennan, & Ullman, 2003; Rogosch, Cicchetti, Toth, & Sheree, 2004; Thompson et al., 2010). Among parents of children with ED, there furthermore appears to be a specific relationship between higher levels of EOI and higher levels of parental anxiety or obsessive-compulsive–related symptoms (Duclos et al., 2014; Rienecke & Richmond, 2017). Psychological distress and caregiver burden are related in parents of children with ED (Coomber & King, 2012). Additionally, there is a positive correlation between patient and carer distress, which in turn mediates the effects of high EE on ED psychopathology (Goddard, Salerno, et al., 2013).

Carer Coping

Several studies suggest that how caregivers cope with such elevated levels of burden and psychological distress affects the relationship of these factors to level of EE. For carers of individuals with ED, adaptive coping is thought to include using humor, positive thinking, acceptance, curiosity, and separation of the illness from the child to manage stress and negative affect (Coomber & King, 2012, 2013; Perkins et al., 2004; Whitney et al., 2005). On the other hand, maladaptive coping is thought to include placing blame on oneself or one's child, feeling helpless, and being overprotective (Coomber & King, 2012). Symptom accommodation is also considered a maladaptive coping mechanism (Rhind et al., 2016; Sepulveda, Kyriacou, & Treasure, 2009). Parents of children with ED tend to use a combination of adaptive and maladaptive coping strategies (Coomber & King, 2013; Perkins et al., 2004). In cross-sectional research, high EE was shown to be associated with higher levels of psychological distress and caregiver burden, and this relationship was mediated by maladaptive coping (Coomber & King, 2012).

When parents hold poorer perceptions of their ill child's difficult behaviors, they are more likely to demonstrate CC (Duclos et al., 2012). Qualitative studies have shown that when their child resists their efforts to influence their eating behaviors, parents find themselves feeling disempowered and engaging in more frequent arguments with their child over food (Fox, Dean, & Whittlesea, 2017; Fox & Whittlesea, 2017). Under such circumstances, parents may become critical or overprotective because they do not understand that difficult behaviors are part of their child's disease, separate from who the child is or how they want to behave (Fox et al., 2017; Fox & Whittlesea, 2017; Whitney et al., 2005; Whitney, Haigh, Weinman, & Treasure, 2007). Alternatively, parents may find themselves becoming more accommodating of ED symptoms due to decreased ability to tolerate the difficult behaviors associated with the ED (Fox et al., 2017). Symptom accommodation on the part of caregivers is positively correlated with elevated EE and negatively correlated with carer skills and social support (Rhind et al., 2016; Sepulveda et al., 2009). Carers' satisfaction with their social support seems to impact the relationship between EE and carer burden and distress, although findings on social support as relate to other ED outcomes have been mixed (Dimitropoulos, Carter, Schachter, & Woodside, 2008; Coomber & King, 2012, 2013). Given that maladaptive coping is a more readily modifiable variable than some of the other factors associated with high EE, it seems to be a prime target for caregiver interventions.

Attributional Style

As described earlier, qualitative research suggests that a carer's ability to effectively manage and cope with their child's ED is influenced by their understanding of the boundaries between their child and the illness and which they believe to be responsible for their child's behavior. This refers to the relative's attributional style, which captures whether they perceive their child's behavior to be caused by something internal, personal, and controllable as opposed to something external, universal, and uncontrollable (Barrowclough & Hooley, 2003). Although this has yet to be quantitatively examined in ED samples, substantial research in the areas of psychotic, mood, anxiety, behavioral, and neurodegenerative disorders indicates that carers' attributions of mental illness-related behaviors are related to their level of EE (Barrowclough & Hooley, 2003; Domínguez-Martínez, Medina-Pradas, Kwapil, & Barrantes-Vidal, 2017; Peris, Yadegar, Asarnow, & Piacentini, 2012; Renshaw, Chambless, & Thorgusen, 2017; Safavi, Berry, & Wearden, 2015). Although these studies were mostly cross-sectional, they provide considerable evidence that high EE relatives are more likely to believe that the patient is personally responsible for their illness-related behaviors. In contrast, low-EE relatives tend to attribute the patient's difficulties to a legitimate, external illness that expresses similar features amongst others it affects.

Understandably, carers who are anxious or fearful about their relatives' illness want to help the patient change. However, those who believe that illness-related behaviors can be voluntarily controlled by the patient are more likely to engage in ineffective social control strategies, such as criticism and blame (Barrowclough & Hooley, 2003; Domínguez-Martínez et al., 2017; Peris et al., 2012; Renshaw et al., 2017; Safavi et al., 2015). There is some evidence to suggest that carers who make more universal and fewer controllable attributions are able to employ more effective approaches, such as expressing empathy and warmth (Barrowclough, Johnston, & Tarrier, 1994; López, Nelson, Snyder, & Mintz, 1999; Weisman, López, Karno, & Jenkins, 1993). Interestingly, the relationship between illness attributions and EE may be influenced by parents' beliefs about non–illness-specific behaviors. In a study of relatives of patients with obsessive-compulsive and panic disorders, participants tended to appropriately attribute disorder related problems to the illness, while non–disorder-related problems were viewed as more controllable (Renshaw et al., 2017). CC and H were associated with controllability attributions for non–disorder-related events, while EOI was associated with illness attributions for non–disorder-related events. In this study, "non–disorder-related events" included issues of anger, irritability, and interpersonal difficulties. While these features are not core symptoms of the disorders of interest, such problems are commonly associated with anxiety and other forms of psychopathology, such as ED. This suggests that clinicians may need to support families in effectively processing attributions of behaviors beyond those that are explicit signs of the illness.

Beyond ED, parents of children with mental health problems do not tend to attribute illness-related difficulties to factors internal to or controllable by themselves (Barrowclough et al., 1994; Brewin, MacCarthy, Duda, & Vaughn, 1991; Tarrier, Barrowclough, Ward, Donaldson, & Burns, 2002; Wendel, Miklowitz, Richards, & George, 2000). However, high EE is associated with elevated levels of guilt and shame among carers of people with mental health difficulties (Bolton et al., 2003; Cherry, Taylor, Brown, Rigby, & Sellwood, 2017). This should be examined in the parents of children with ED, as they have historically shouldered inaccurate and inappropriate responsibility for their children's' ED (Le Grange, Lock, Loeb, & Nicholls, 2010). Thus, parents of children with ED may experience personal responsibility and blame differently than parents of children with other psychological disorders.

Gender

Differences between maternal and paternal EE and their relationship to other important variables have been noted throughout this chapter. Indeed, it seems that there are differences between mothers and fathers regarding EE in the context of ED (Duclos et al., 2014; Rienecke et al.,

2017). Some have found that mothers demonstrate higher CC (Allan et al., 2018; Duclos et al., 2012; Schwarte et al., 2017) and EOI (Allan et al., 2018; Anastasiadou, Sepulveda, Parks, Cuellar-Flores, & Graell, 2016; Blondin et al., 2019; Duclos et al., 2012; Kyriacou et al., 2008; Le Grange et al., 2011; Rienecke & Richmond, 2017; Rhind et al., 2016; Schwarte et al., 2017). Mothers also demonstrate higher levels of positive features of EE, such as PR and W (Duclos et al., 2012). However, there do not appear to be consistent differences in overall levels of EE between mothers and fathers (Di Paola et al., 2010; Duclos et al., 2014; Moulds et al., 2000), and maternal and paternal EE tend to be correlated (Blondin et al., 2019; Duclos et al., 2012; Rhind et al., 2016).

Other factors that have been associated with high EE may account for the differences in EE correlates across mothers and fathers. For example, mothers typically have much more contact with the ill child and spend significantly more time involved in caring tasks (Anastasiadou et al., 2016; Duclos et al., 2012; Kyriacou et al., 2008; Rhind et al., 2016), which is associated with elevated EE. This difference in contact hours may also account for why maternal EE appears to have a greater impact on family functioning and treatment outcomes (Eisler et al., 2007; Rienecke et al., 2016). As described earlier, parental anxiety and depression are positively correlated with high EE, and mothers of children with ED tend to experience higher levels of such psychological distress (Kyriacou et al., 2008; Rhind et al., 2016; Schwarte et al., 2017). This, too, could be related to having more contact with the ill child or socialized differences in gender roles and expressions. It is important to remember that the bulk of the research on EE in parents of children with ED is limited, as it is predicated on the assumption that parents are usually cis-gendered heterosexual white couples.

Family Factors Associated With Level of EE

As compared with patient and parent-related variables, there has been relatively less attention paid to aspects of the broader family context that might be associated with level of EE in ED populations. There have been limited findings regarding the socioeconomic status (SES) of the family, with one study showing that higher SES groups are more likely to demonstrate high EE, particularly CC (Szmukler et al., 1985).

Additionally, there is some evidence that non-white parents tended to show relatively lower levels of W and PR than white parents (Hoste et al., 2012; Hoste & Le Grange, 2008). Research from other domains of psychopathology suggest that there is no relationship between EE and demographic variables such as SES or ethnicity, suggesting that EE is not a proxy for general demographic risk (Baker, Heller, & Henker, 2000; Boger et al., 2008; Stubbe, Zahner, Goldstein, & Leckman, 1993). Cultural differences in expressed emotion are reviewed in greater depth elsewhere in this text (see Chapter 8).

There has been minimal research examining how family structure and functioning might relate to level of caregiver EE in the context of ED. In a study of adults with BN, families were shown to have high levels of conflict and lower levels of organization when caregivers had high EE (Hedlund et al., 2003). One study suggested that the presence of siblings might reduce maternal W and EOI, but no such effect was found for fathers (Rienecke, Sim, et al., 2016). There has been little research on parental separation and EE as pertains to ED. One study found that the family's status as intact or separated had no impact on EE (Schwarte et al., 2017). Another study reported that fathers from intact families had higher W and lower CC than fathers from separated families (Rienecke, Sim, et al., 2016). In this same study, mothers from intact families tended to have lower CC but also lower PR. Studies of children with other forms of psychopathology suggest that high-EE families tend to experience greater levels of family conflict, marital problems, and poor communication (Boger et al., 2008; Hibbs, Hamburger, Kruesi, & Lenane, 1993; Kymalainen & Weisman de Mamani, 2008; Stubbe et al., 1993; Wearden, Tarrier, Barrowclough, Zastowny, & Rahill, 2000). Widening the lens to capture more information about the broader family context could be useful, particularly given the preeminence of family-based approaches to treating ED.

Conclusions

In general, raising children is not experienced as an easy task by most parents. One does not receive any prior training in parenting, and the most influential parenting examples are one's own parents. This makes it all the more understandable that coping with a child with a serious illness such as an ED offers an extra challenge to most parents. EDs, specifically AN, engender anxiety in all parents and perceived powerlessness in many. As clinicians, we may never see the parents who respond swiftly and decisively to the first signs of weight loss in their child.

In contrast to the body of evidence linking parental EE attitudes to outcome in ED, we still have limited insight into the factors associated with high and low EE. Most of the studies investigating these factors are cross-sectional in nature, and the results from different studies are rarely consistent. There is some evidence to suggest that illness-related behaviors that are perceived as difficult to control by parents, such as dieting, bingeing, purging, apathy, and hopelessness due to depression, are associated with higher levels of EE, especially when these behaviors persist, sometimes for many years. Interest in the child's EE as a potential predictor of outcome has surfaced only recently (Hoste, Lebow, & Le Grange, 2015; Rienecke, Lebow, et al., 2017). Individual attitudes develop prospectively in the interactions between family members. Developmentally appropriate teen behaviors mixed with the strong influence of an ED on child behavior may easily interact in a circular fashion with parental coping style and perceived burden, resulting in psychological distress in all family members.

In the various forms of family-based therapy, one aims to modify the attitudes and behaviors of family members to enhance effective age- and role-appropriate collaboration between them to overcome the ED (Hughes, Sawyer, Loeb, & Le Grange, 2015; Lock & Le Grange, 2013). Parents with a high perceived burden of care or high levels of psychological distress (sometimes exacerbated by their own history) and children with a high-EE attitude towards their parents warrant extra attention in therapy.

References

Allan, E., Le Grange, D., Sawyer, S. M., McLean, L. A., & Hughes, E. K. (2018). Parental expressed emotion during two forms of family-based treatment for adolescent anorexia nervosa. *European Eating Disorders Review*, *26*, 46–52. doi:10.1002/erv.2564

Anastasiadou, D., Medina-Pradas, C., Sepulveda, A. R., & Treasure, J. (2014). A systematic review of family caregiving in eating disorders. *Eating Behaviors*, *15*(3), 464–477. doi:10.1016/j.eatbeh.2014.06.001

Anastasiadou, D., Sepulveda, A. R., Parks, M., Cuellar-Flores, I., & Graell, M. (2016). The relationship between dysfunctional family patterns and symptom severity among adolescent patients with eating disorders: A gender-specific approach. *Women & Health*, *56*, 695–712. doi:10.1080/03630242.2015.1118728

Baker, B. L., Heller, T. L., & Henker, B. (2000). Expression emotion, parenting stress, and adjustment in mothers of young children with behavior problems. *Journal of Child Psychology and Psychology and Other Allied Disciplines*, *41*, 907–915. doi:10.1111/1469-7610.00678

Barrowclough, C., & Hooley, J. M. (2003). Attributions and expressed emotion: A review. *Clinical Psychology Review*, *23*, 849–880. doi:10.1016/S0272-7358(03)00075-8

Barrowclough, C., Johnston, M., & Tarrier, N. (1994). Attributions, expressed emotion, and patient relapse: An attributional model of relatives' response to schizophrenic illness. *Behavior Therapy*, *25*, 67–88. doi:10.1016/S0005-7894(05)80146-7

Blair, C., Freeman, C., & Cull, A. (1995). The families of anorexia nervosa and cystic fibrosis patients. *Psychological Medicine*, *25*, 985–993. doi:10.1017/S0033291700037478

Blondin, S., Meilleur, D., Taddeo, D., & Frappier, J. (2019). Caregiving experience and expressed emotion among parents of adolescents suffering from anorexia nervosa following illness onset. *Eating Disorders*, np. doi:10.1080/10640266.2018.1553431

Boger, K. D., Tompson, M. C., Briggs-Gowan, M. J., Pavlis, L. E., & Carter, A. S. (2008). Parental expressed emotion toward children: Prediction from early family functioning. *Journal of Family Psychology*, *22*, 784–788. doi:10.1037/a0013251

Bolton, C., Calam, R., Barrowclough, C., Peters, S., Roberts, J., Wearden, A., & Morris, J. (2003). Expressed emotion, attributions, and depression in mothers of children with problem behavior. *Journal of Child Psychology and Psychiatry*, *44*, 242–254. doi:10.1111/1469-7610.00117

Brewin, C. R., MacCarthy, B., Duda, K., & Vaughn, C. E. (1991). Attributions and expressed emotion in the relatives of patients with schizophrenia. *Journal of Abnormal Psychology*, *100*, 546–554. doi:10.1037/0021-843x.100.4.546

Brown, G. W., Birley, J. L., & Wing, J. K. (1972). Influence of family life on the course of schizophrenic disorders: A replication. *British Journal of Psychiatry*, *121*, 241–258. doi:10.1192/bjp.121.3.241

Cherry, M. G., Taylor, P. J., Brown, S. L., Rigby, J. W., & Sellwood, W. (2017). Guilt, shame and expressed emotion in carers of people with long-term mental health difficulties: A systematic review. *Psychiatry Research*, *249*, 139–151. doi:10.1016/j.psychres.2016.12.056

Christiansen, H., Oades, R. D., Psychogiou, L., Hauffa, B. P., & Sonuga-Barke, E. J. (2010). Does the cortisol response to stress mediate the link between expressed emotion and oppositional behavior in Attention-Deficit/Hyperactivity Disorder (ADHD)? *Behavioral and Brain Functions*, *6*, 45. doi:10.1186/1744-9081-6-45

Coomber, K., & King, R. M. (2012). Coping strategies and social support as predictors and mediators of eating disorder carer burden and psychological distress. *Social Psychiatry and Psychiatric Epidemiology*, *47*, 789–796. doi:10.1007/s00127-011-0384-6

Coomber, K., & King, R. M. (2013). A longitudinal examination of burden and psychological distress in carers of people with an eating disorder. *Social Psychiatry and Psychiatric Epidemiology*, *48*, 163–171. doi:10.1007/s00127-012-0524-7

Dimitropoulos, G., Carter, J., Schachter, R., & Woodside, D. B. (2008). Predictors of family functioning in carers of individuals with anorexia nervosa. *International Journal of Eating Disorders*, *41*, 739–747. doi:10.1002/eat.20562

Di Paola, F., Faravelli, C., & Ricca, V. (2010). Expressed emotion in anorexia nervosa, bulimia nervosa, and binge-eating disorder. *Comprehensive Psychiatry*, *51*, 401–405. doi:10.1016/j.comppsych.2009.10.002

Domínguez-Martínez, T., Medina-Pradas, C., Kwapil, T. R., & Barrantes-Vidal, N. (2017). Relatives' expressed emotion, distress and attributions in clinical high-risk and recent onset of psychosis. *Psychiatry Research, 247*, 323–329. doi:10.1016/j.psychres.2016.11.048

Duclos, J., Dorard, G., Berthoz, S., Curt, F., Faucher, S., Falissard, B., & Godart, N. (2014). Expressed emotion in anorexia nervosa: What is inside the "black box"? *Comprehensive Psychiatry, 55*, 71–79. doi:10.1016/j.comppsych.2013.10.002

Duclos, J., Maria, A.-S., Dorard, G., Curt, F., Apfel, A., Vibert, S., . . . Godart, N. (2013). Bonding and expressed emotion: Two interlinked concepts? *Psychopathology, 46*, 404–412. doi:10.1159/000345405

Duclos, J., Vibert, S., Mattar, L., & Godart, N. (2012). Expressed emotion in families of patients with eating disorders: A review of the literature. *Current Psychiatry Reviews, 8*, 183–202. doi:10.2174/157340012800792975

Eisler, I., Dare, C., Hodes, M., Russell, G., Dodge, E., & Le Grange, D. (2000). Family therapy for adolescent anorexia nervosa: The results of a controlled comparison of two family interventions. *Journal of Child Psychology and Psychiatry, 41*, 727–736. doi:10.1111/1469-7610.00660

Eisler, I., Simic, M., Russell, G. F. M., & Dare, C. (2007). A randomised controlled treatment trial of two forms of family therapy in adolescent anorexia nervosa: A five-year follow-up. *Journal of Child Psychology and Psychiatry, 48*, 552–560. doi:10.1111/j.1469-7610.2007.01726.x

Fox, J. R. E., Dean, M., & Whittlesea, A. (2017). The experience of caring for or living with an individual with an eating disorder: A meta-synthesis of qualitative studies. *Clinical Psychology and Psychotherapy, 24*, 103–125. doi:10.1002/cpp.1984

Fox, J. R. E., & Whittlesea, A. (2017). Accommodation of symptoms in anorexia nervosa: A qualitative study. *Clinical Psychology and Psychotherapy, 24*, 488–599. doi:10.1002/cpp.2020

Goddard, E., Hibbs, R., Raenker, S., Salerno, L., Areclus, J., Boughton, N., . . . Treasure, J. (2013). A multi-centre cohort study of short term outcomes of hospital treatment for anorexia nervosa in the UK. *BMC Psychiatry, 13*, 287. doi:10.1186/1471-244X-13-287

Goddard, E., Salerno, L., Hibbs, R., Raenker, S., Naumann, U., Areclus, J., . . . Treasure, J. (2013). Empirical examination of the interpersonal maintenance model of anorexia nervosa. *International Journal of Eating Disorders, 46*, 867–874. doi:10.1002/eat.22172

Hedlund, S., Fichter, M. M., Quadflieg, N., & Brandl, C. (2003). Expressed emotion, family environment, and parental bonding in bulimia nervosa: A 6-year investigation. *Eating and Weight Disorders, 8*, 26–35. doi:10.1007/BF03324986

Hibbs, E. D., Hamburger, S. D., Kruesi, M. J., & Lenane, M. (1993). Factors affecting expressed emotion in parents of ill and normal children. *American Journal of Orthopsychiatry, 63*, 103–112. doi:10.1037/h0079395

Hibbs, E. D., Hamburger, S. D., Lenane, M., Rapoport, J. L., Kruesi, M. J., Keysor, C. S., & Goldstein, M. J. (1991). Determinants of expressed emotion in families of disturbed and normal children. *Journal of Child Psychology and Psychiatry and Allied Disciplines, 32*, 757–770. doi:10.1111/j.1469-7610.1991.tb01900.x

Hibbs, E. D., Zahn, T. P., Hamburger, S. D., Kruesi, M. M., & Rapoport, J. L. (1992). Parental expressed emotion and psychophysiological reactivity in disturbed and normal children. *British Journal of Psychiatry, 160*, 504–510. doi:10.1192/bjp.160.4.504

Hooley, J. M., Gruber, S. A., Parker, H. A., Guillaumot, J., Rogowska, J., & Yurgelun-Tudd, D. A. (2009). Cortico-limbic response to personally challenging emotional stimuli after complete recovery from depression. *Psychiatry Research, 172*, 83–91. doi:10.1016/j.pscychresns.2009.02.001

Hooley, J. M., Gruber, S. A., Scott, L. A., Hiller, J. B., & Yurgelun-Todd, D. A. (2005). Activation in dorsolateral prefrontal cortex in response to maternal criticism and praise in recovered depressed and healthy control participants. *Biological Psychiatry, 57*, 809–812. doi:10.1016/j.biopsych.2005.01.012

Hoste, R. R., Labuschagne, Z., Lock, J., & Le Grange, D. (2012). Cultural variability in expressed emotion among families of adolescents with anorexia nervosa. *International Journal of Eating Disorders, 45*, 142–145. doi:10.1002/eat.20888

Hoste, R. R., Lebow, J., & Le Grange, D. (2015). A bidirectional examination of expressed emotion among families of adolescents with bulimia nervosa. *International Journal of Eating Disorders, 48*, 249–252. doi:10.1002/eat.22306

Hoste, R. R., & Le Grange, D. (2008). Expressed emotion among white and ethnic minority families of adolescents with bulimia nervosa. *European Eating Disorders Review, 16*, 395–400. doi:10.1002/erv.856

Hughes, E. K., Sawyer, S. M., Loeb, K. L., & Le Grange, D. (2015). Parent-focused treatment. In K. L. Loeb, D. Le Grange, & J. Lock (Eds.), *Family therapy for adolescent eating and weight disorders: New applications* (pp. 59–71). New York, NY: Routledge.

Kaye, W. H., Fudge, J. L., & Paulus, M. (2009). New insights into symptoms and neurocircuit function of anorexia nervosa. *Nature Reviews Neuroscience, 10*, 573–584. doi:10.1038/nrn2682

Klump, W., Bulik, C. M., Pollice, C., Halmi, K. A., Fichter, M. M., Berrettini, W. H., . . . Kaye, W. H. (2000). Temperament and character in women with anorexia nervosa. *Journal of Nervous and Mental Disease, 188*, 559–567. doi:10.1097/00005053-200009000-00001

Kymalainen, J. A., & Weisman de Mamani, A. G. (2008). Expressed emotion, communication deviance, and culture in families of patients with schizophrenia: A review of the literature. *Cultural Diversity and Ethnic Minority Psychology, 14*, 85–91. doi:10.1037/1099-9809.14.2.85

Kyriacou, O., Treasure, J., & Schmidt, U. (2008). Expression emotion in eating disorders assessed via self-report: An examination of factors associated with expressed emotion in carers of people with anorexia nervosa in comparison to control families. *International Journal of Eating Disorders, 41*, 37–46. doi:10.1002/eat

Le Grange, D., Eisler, I., Dare, C., & Hodes, M. (1992). Family criticism and self-starvation: A study of expressed emotion. *Journal of Family Therapy, 14*, 177–192. doi:10.1046/j.1992.00451.x

Le Grange, D., Eisler, I., Dare, C., & Russell, G. F. M. (1992). Evaluation of family treatments in adolescent anorexia nervosa: A pilot study. *International Journal of Eating Disorders, 12*, 347–357. doi:10.1002/1098-108X(199212)12:4<347::AID-EAT2260120402>3.0.CO;2-W

Le Grange, D., Hoste, R., Lock, J., & Bryson, S. W. (2011). Parental expressed emotion of adolescents with anorexia nervosa: Outcome in family-based treatment. *International Journal of Eating Disorders, 44*, 731–734. doi:10.1002/eat.20877

Le Grange, D., Lock, J., Loeb, K. L., & Nicholls, D. (2010). Academy for eating disorders position paper: The role of the family in eating disorders. *International Journal of Eating Disorders, 43*, 1–5. doi:10.1002/eat.20751

Lock, J., & Le Grange, D. (2013). *Treatment manual for anorexia nervosa: A family-based approach* (2nd ed.). New York, NY: Guilford Press.

López, S. R., Nelson, K. A., Snyder, K. S., & Mintz, J. (1999). Attributions and affective reactions of family members and course of schizophrenia. *Journal of Abnormal Psychology, 108*, 307–314. doi:10.1037/0021-843X.108.2.307

McCarty, C. A., & Weisz, J. R. (2002). Correlated of expressed emotion in mothers of clinically-referred youth: An examination of the five-minute speech sample. *Journal of Child Psychology and Psychiatry and Allied Disciplines, 43*, 759–768. doi:10.1111/1469-7610.00090

Medina-Pradas, C., Blas Navarro, J., López, S. R., Grau, A., & Obiols, J. E. (2011). Dyadic view of expressed emotion, stress, and eating disorder psychopathology. *Appetite, 57*, 743–748. doi:10.1016/j.appet.2011.08.016

Meyer, C., Leung, N., Barry, L., & De Feo, D. (2010). Emotion and eating psychopathology: Links with attitudes toward emotional expression among young women. *International Journal of Eating Disorders, 43*, 187–189. doi:10.1002/eat.20659

Moulds, M. L., Touyz, S. W., Schotte, D., Beumont, P. J. V., Griffiths, R., Russell, J., & Charles, M. (2000). Perceived expressed emotion in the siblings and parents of hospitalized patients with anorexia nervosa. *Eating Disorders, 27*, 288–296. doi:10.1002/(SICI)1098-108X(200004)27:3<288::AID-EAT5>3.0.CO;2-7

Munsch, S., Dremmel, D., Kurz, S., De Albuquerque, J., Meyer, A. H., & Hilbert, A. (2017). Influence of parental expressed emotions on children's emotional eating via children's negative urgency. *European Eating Disorders Review, 25*, 36–41. doi:10.1002/erv.2489

Nelson, D. R., Hammen, C., Brennan, P. A., & Ullman, J. B. (2003). The impact of maternal depression on adolescent adjustment: The role of expressed emotion. *Journal of Consulting and Clinical Psychology, 71*, 935–944. doi:10.1037/0022-006X.71.5.935

Peris, T. S., & Miklowitz, D. J. (2015). Parental expressed emotion and youth psychopathology: New directions for an old construct. *Child Psychiatry & Human Development, 46*, 863–873. doi:10.1007/s10578-014-0526-7

Peris, T. S., Yadegar, M., Asarnow, J. R., & Piacentini, J. (2012). Pediatric obsessive compulsive disorder: Family climate as a predictor of treatment outcome. *Journal of Obsessive-Compulsive and Related Disorders, 1*, 267–273. doi:10.1016/j.jocrd.2012.07.003

Perkins, S., Winn, S., Murray, J., Murphy, R., & Schmidt, U. (2004). A qualitative study of the experience of caring for a person with bulimia nervosa, Part 1: The emotional impact of caring. *International Journal of Eating Disorders, 36*, 256–268. doi:10.1002/eat.20067

Renshaw, K. D., Chambless, D. L., & Thorgusen, S. (2017). Expressed emotion and attributions in relatives of patients with obsessive-compulsive disorder and panic disorder. *Journal of Nervous and Mental Disease, 205*, 294–299. doi:10.1097/NMD.0000000000000636

Rhind, C., Salerno, L., Hibbs, R., Micali, N., Schmidt, U., Gowers, S., . . . Treasure, J. (2016). The objective and subjective caregiving burden and caregiving behaviours of parents of adolescents with anorexia nervosa. *European Eating Disorders Review, 24*, 310–319. doi:10.1002/erv.2442

Rienecke, R. D., Accurso, E. C., Lock, J., & Le Grange, D. (2016). Expressed emotion, family functioning, and treatment outcome for adolescents with anorexia nervosa. *European Eating Disorders Review, 24*, 43–51. doi:10.1002/erv.2389

Rienecke, R. D., Lebow, J., Lock, J., & Le Grange, D. (2017). Family profiles of expressed emotion in adolescent patients with anorexia nervosa and their parents. *Journal of Clinical Child & Adolescent Psychology, 46*, 428–436. doi:10.1080/15374416.2015.1030755

Rienecke, R. D., & Richmond, R. L. (2017). Psychopathology and expressed emotion in parents of patients with eating disorders: Relation to patient symptom severity. *Eating Disorders, 25*, 318–329. doi:10.1080/10640266.2017.1289795

Rienecke, R. D., Sim, L., Lock, J., & Le Grange, D. (2016). Patterns of expressed emotion in adolescent eating disorders. *Journal of Child Psychology and Psychiatry, 57*, 1407–1413. doi:10.1111/jcpp.12594

Rogosch, F. A., Cicchetti, D., Toth, S. L., & Sheree, L. (2004). Expressed emotion in multiple subsystems of the families of toddlers with depressed mothers. *Development and Psychopathology, 16*, 689–709. doi:10.1017/S0954579404004730P

Safavi, R., Berry, K., & Wearden, A. (2015). Expressed emotion in relatives of persons with dementia: A systematic review and meta-analysis. *Aging & Mental Health*, *21*, 113–124. doi:10.1080/13607863.2015.1111863

Santonastaso, P., Saccon, D., & Favaro, A. (1997). Burden and psychiatric symptoms on key relatives of patients with eating disorders: A preliminary study. *Eating and Weight Disorders*, *2*, 44–48. doi:10.1007/BF03339949

Schmidt, R., Tetzlaff, A., & Hilbert, A. (2015). Perceived expressed emotion in adolescents with binge-eating disorder. *Journal of Abnormal Child Psychology*, *43*, 1369–1377. doi:10.1007/s10802-015-0015-x

Schwarte, R., Timmesfeld, N., Dempfle, A., Krei, M., Egberts, K., Jaite, C., . . . Bühren, K. (2017). Expressed emotions and depressive symptoms in caregivers of adolescents with first-onset anorexia nervosa: A long-term investigation over 2.5 years. *European Eating Disorders Review*, *25*, 44–51. doi:10.1002/erv.2490

Sepulveda, A. R., Kyriacou, O., & Treasure, J. (2009). Development and validation of the Accommodation and Enabling Scale for Eating Disorders (AESED) for caregivers in eating disorders. *BMC Health Services Research*, *9*, 171. doi:10.1186/1472-6963-9-171.

Sepulveda, A. R., Todd, G., Whitaker, W., Grover, M., Stahl, D., & Treasure, J. (2010). Expressed emotion in relatives of patients with eating disorders following skills training program. *International Journal of Eating Disorders*, *43*, 603–610. doi:10.1002/eat.20749

Stubbe, D. E., Zahner, G. E. P., Goldstein, M. J., & Leckman, J. F. (1993). Diagnostic specificity of a brief measure of expressed emotion: A community study of children. *Journal of Child Psychology and Psychiatry*, *34*, 139–154. doi:10.1111/j.1469-7610.1993.tb00976.x

Szmukler, G. I., Eisler, I., Russell, G. F., & Dare, C. (1985). Anorexia nervosa, parental "expressed emotion" and dropping out of treatment. *British Journal of Psychiatry*, *147*, 265–271. doi:10.1192/bjp.147.3.265

Tarrier, N., Barrowclough, C., Ward, J., Donaldson, C., & Burns, A. (2002). Expressed emotion and attributions in the carers of patients with Alzheimer's disease. *Journal of Abnormal Psychology*, *111*, 340–349. doi:10.1037/0021-843x.111.2.340

Thompson, M. C., Pierre, C. B., Boger, K. D., McKowen, J. W., Chan, P. T., & Freed, R. D. (2010). Maternal depression, maternal expressed emotion, and youth psychopathology. *Journal of Abnormal Child Psychology*, *38*, 105–117. doi:10.1007/s10802-009-9349-6

van Furth, E. F., van Strien, D. C., Martina, L. M., van Son, M. J., Hendrickx, J. J., & van Engeland, H. (1996). Expressed emotion and the prediction of outcome in adolescent eating disorders. *International Journal of Eating Disorders*, *20*, 19–31. doi:10.1002/(SICI)1098-108X(199607)20:1<19::AID-EAT3>3.0.CO;2-7

Wearden, A. J., Tarrier, N., Barrowclough, C., Zastowny, T. R., & Rahill, A. A. (2000). A review of expressed emotion research in health care. *Clinical Psychology Review*, *20*, 633–666. doi:10.1016/S0272-7358(99)00008-2

Weisman, A., López, S. R., Karno, M., & Jenkins, J. (1993). An attributional analysis of expressed emotion in Mexican-American families with schizophrenia. *Journal of Abnormal Psychology*, *102*, 601–606. doi:10.1037/0021-843x.102.4.601

Wendel, J. S., Miklowitz, D. J., Richard, J. A., & George, E. L. (2000). Expressed emotion and attributions in the relatives of bipolar patients: An analysis of problem solving interactions. *Journal of Abnormal Psychology*, *109*, 792–796. doi:10.1037/0021-843X.109.4.792

Whitney, J., Haigh, R., Weinman, J., & Treasure, J. (2007). Caring for people with eating disorders: Factors associated with psychological distress and negative caregiving appraisals in carers of people with eating disorders. *British Journal of Clinical Psychology*, *46*, 413–428. doi:10.1348/014466507X173781

Whitney, J., Murray, J., Gavan, K., Todd, G., Whitaker, W., & Treasure, J. (2005). Experience of caring for someone with anorexia nervosa: A qualitative study. *British Journal of Psychiatry*, *187*, 444–449. doi:10.1192/bjp.187.5.444

Winn, S., Perkins, S., Walwyn, R., Schmidt, U., Eisler, I., Treasure, J., . . . Yi, I. (2007). Predictors of mental health problems and negative caregiving experiences in carers of adolescents with bulimia nervosa. *International Journal of Eating Disorders*, *40*, 171–178. doi:10.1002/eat.20347

Zabala, M. J., Macdonald, P., & Treasure, J. (2009). Appraisal of caregiving burden, expressed emotion and psychological distress in families of people with eating disorders: A systematic review. *European Eating Disorders Review*, *17*, 338–349. doi:10.1002/erv.925

10

Future Directions in Expressed Emotion

Renee D. Rienecke and Gina Dimitropoulos

Introduction

This book demonstrates the wealth of research on expressed emotion (EE) in eating disorders over the past 30 years. However, gaps in research have been noted by the contributors, pointing to the many opportunities for future researchers to further advance our knowledge and understanding of EE within the eating disorder context. For instance, there is a need for intervention research specifically designed for affected individuals and their caregivers, rather than focusing exclusively on family interventions, which may not always be feasible, sufficient, or appropriate (see Chapter 2). Intervention research is needed to facilitate a reduction of Critical Comments and an increase in warmth during different stages of the illness, different developmental stages of the individual with the eating disorder, and illness trajectory (short duration versus chronic illness). In addition, improvement of current family interventions, taking into consideration factors such as neurobiology, temperament, and emotion regulation, may also be useful, as will developing an understanding of why separated family therapy may be more preferable than conjoint family therapy when working with families with high levels of EE (see Chapters 3, 5, and 7). To ease comparison across studies, consistent use of well-validated measures of EE is important, which may necessitate the development of new EE measures or adaptation of existing measures and scoring criteria, particularly in regard to Emotional Overinvolvement (EOI) and its application to children and adolescents (see Chapters 3, 4, and 5).

Less research has been conducted on patients with bulimia nervosa (BN) than anorexia nervosa (AN), with mixed findings regarding the relative levels of EE in these different diagnostic groups (see Chapter 6). Additional research in this area will be useful, including a better understanding of possible reasons behind different levels of EE in families with an individual with AN versus BN, as well as gathering more information on EE among those with binge eating disorder (BED), avoidant/restrictive food intake disorder (ARFID), and other specified feeding or eating disorder (OSFED). Much also remains to be learned about cultural differences in EE (see Chapter 8), particularly the various ways in which high EE can be expressed and tolerated based on the cultural context. Other issues of diversity must also be further investigated in the context of EE. For example, the majority of research on EE has predominantly focused on mothers or heterosexual parents. Future research is needed to understand different family structures, including sole support parents, blended families, and parents who are members of a sexual minority group. Finally, further research is needed on factors that differentiate high- from low-EE families (see Chapter 9), with particular emphasis on a better understanding of low-EE families. Other more focused areas for future research that have been identified throughout this volume are reviewed as potential research priorities.

Mechanisms of Action in Expressed Emotion

EE has been found to be a robust predictor of treatment dropout, outcome, and relapse across a range of psychiatric and medical disorders (Butzlaff & Hooley, 1998; Wearden, Tarrier, Barrowclough, Zastowny, & Rahill, 2000). However, understanding of the theory behind EE and its mechanisms of action has lagged behind outcome research, leading some to refer to EE as a "black box" (Jenkins & Karno, 1992). One fruitful area for future research would be further elucidation of the ways in which high EE leads to poor outcomes for patients in eating disorders, thereby informing more targeted therapeutic interventions for patients and their families, ultimately improving clinical outcomes for these patients.

Hooley and Gotlib (2000) propose a diathesis-stress model as one way to conceptualize the EE-outcomes pathway. Intriguingly, they suggest that the mechanisms of action, in terms of how high EE leads to poor outcomes, may differ depending on the disorder. For example, Brown and colleagues proposed that patients with schizophrenia are highly sensitive to environmental stressors and may find high-EE relatives to be overstimulating (Brown, Birley, & Wing, 1972). Early psychophysiological studies found that patients with schizophrenia showed an increase in blood pressure when a high-EE relative entered the room, whereas patients showed a decrease in the frequency of non-specific skin conductance responses when low-EE relatives entered the room (Tarrier, Vaughn, Lader, & Leff, 1979), suggesting that patients with schizophrenia are physiologically aroused around relatives who are high in EE, while they may find the presence of low-EE relatives to be calming. Other early studies showed similar results (Altorfer, Käsermann, & Hirsbrunner, 1998; Sturgeon, Turpin, Kuipers, Berkowitz, & Leff, 1984), ultimately leading to hypotheses that stressful events lead to an increase in cortisol, which in turn can stimulate the dopaminergic system, leading to an increase in symptoms of schizophrenia (Davis, Kahn, Ko, & Davidson, 1991). Future studies could investigate whether similar increases in cortisol or other biomarkers are found among those with eating disorders and whether this in turn may lead to a worsening of eating disorder symptoms.

A related conceptualization of EE is as a form of "toxic family stress" (Peris & Miklowitz, 2015), whereby caregivers react negatively to the presence of psychiatric illness in their child, creating an environment that is physiologically arousing and stressful. Similar to findings in adults with schizophrenia, studies have found that high parental EE is linked to elevated levels of salivary cortisol in youth with ADHD (Christiansen, Oades, Psychogious, Hauffa, & Sonuga-Barke, 2010) and to elevated baseline stress, measured by skin conductance, for youth with obsessive-compulsive disorder (Hibbs, Zahn, Hamburger, & Kruesi, 1992). Elevated stress can be associated with increased symptoms (Humphreys et al., 2019; Morgado, Freitas, Bessa, Sousa, & Cerqueira, 2013), which in turn can increase negative interpersonal interactions, then leading to increased Criticism, Hostility, or EOI on the part of caregivers, creating a vicious cycle between patients and caregivers. Toxic family stress may play a role in worsening symptoms in patients with eating disorders, perhaps particularly for those with AN, who have been shown to be highly sensitive to punishment (Jappe et al., 2011). This may be why studies of EE in AN have found poor outcome associated with the presence of as few as one critical comment (e.g., Rienecke, Accurso, Lock, & Le Grange, 2016), as opposed to studies of patients with schizophrenia, with whom the cutoff for Critical Comments has historically been six (Vaughn & Leff, 1976). Future research is needed to further investigate the possible role of toxic family stress in eating disorders.

Different mechanisms of action leading to poor treatment outcome are proposed for patients with depression. The information-processing style of individuals with depression is characterized in part by difficulties in disengaging from negative stimuli, tendencies to misinterpret stimuli, and improved memory for negative material (Beck & Clark, 1988; Foland-Ross & Gotlib, 2012). This may cause patients to be particularly attuned to and to remember Critical Comments from relatives, thus increasing their depressive symptoms. Hooley and Gotlib (2000) suggest that this may be why two or three Critical Comments from family members have been found to be associated with relapse, as opposed to the cutoff of six Critical Comments that is usually used in schizophrenia research.

Patients with borderline personality disorder (BPD), on the other hand, have been shown to respond to high EE differently than patients with schizophrenia or depression. A study of 35 inpatients with BPD found that caregiver Criticism and Hostility were not related to relapse and that *high* EOI was predictive of better outcome and not being rehospitalized (Hooley & Hoffman, 1999). While it is unclear why this may be, it does suggest that reactions to EE differ depending on the diagnosis of the patient and that the mechanisms leading to poor outcome and relapse may vary across diagnoses. In the eating disorders field, there is limited evidence to suggest that patients with AN and patients with BN may respond differently to high parental EE (Hoste, Lebow, & Le Grange, 2015; Rienecke, Lebow, Lock, & Le Grange, 2017), but further research is needed to investigate this.

Understanding the mechanisms involved in outcomes can lead to the development of more effective treatments. For example, common elements of family treatment for schizophrenia involve psychoeducation and work on structured problem solving within the family (Caqueo-Urízar, Rus-Calafell, Urzúa, Escudero, & Gutiérrez-Maldonado, 2015). Reducing interpersonal tensions may decrease autonomic arousal for the patient, in turn reducing symptoms (Hooley & Gotlib, 2000). Cognitive restructuring may be more appropriate for patients with depression. Future research in the field of eating disorders should seek to determine the pathways whereby high EE leads to poor outcome and treatment dropout for these particular patients, thus enabling clinicians and researchers to take this into consideration when developing and choosing treatment interventions. For example, treatment may be improved by adding psychoeducation for parents about the temperament of patients with AN as well as the nature of AN, perhaps with particular attention to parental attributional style (see Chapter 9), and correcting misperceptions about the disorder. Addressing attributions about ED behavior is recommended as part of family-based treatment (Lock & Le Grange, 2013) and may be useful in other forms of treatment involving caregivers, both for the treatment of eating disorders and more broadly for other psychiatric diagnoses.

Integrated Theoretical Framework

An integrated theoretical framework has been proposed that considers the neurobiology, temperament, cognitive appraisal, and emotion regulation of patients with eating disorders (described in Chapter 3). This theoretical model provides the groundwork for innovative research to test this model in EE in eating disorders. For instance, there is a need to understand how affect regulation contributes to varying levels of EE in caregivers of individuals with eating disorders. Preliminary findings suggest that parental mental health concerns and difficulties regulating affect during times of distress may contribute to heightened EE in individuals with bipolar disorder (Millman, Weintraub, & Miklowitz, 2018). If emotional distress is correlated with EE, interventions may need to be developed and tested to support caregivers during acute stages of the illness or the occurrence of a relapse in eating disorders.

EE Across Stages of Illness

Caregivers of people with eating disorders have reported the need for interventions to assist them with their distress, the burdens and demands of caring, and managing symptoms and navigating services for their loved one (Haigh & Treasure, 2003). A meta-analysis of caregiver interventions showed a reduction in EE by targeting psychosocial distress and burden for a wide range of carers of those with eating disorders (Hibbs et al., 2015). A recent study assessed whether a short intervention (two 2.5-hour sessions) would be effective at influencing caregiver burden, EE, and accommodation levels in carers compared with a waitlist control group. Although this brief intervention lead to some improvements in caregiver burden, no changes were found in EE. To date, caregiver interventions for eating disorders have yielded conflicting results in reducing EE (Dimitropoulos et al., 2019; Pépin & King, 2013). Research is needed to identify whether distinct types of interventions (educational, skills based, or a combination of the two) might be required for individuals and their families at different stages of the illness. For instance, are briefer psychoeducation interventions the first line of treatment for carers of a loved one presenting for treatment for the first time for emerging or new symptoms of AN or BN? Schwarte et al. (2017) found that EE was heightened at the initial phase of treatment and then declined over treatment and peaked again for those who relapsed two years following treatment. This study suggests that some caregivers of those with persistent symptoms may require communication and problem-solving groups or individual sessions to assist with warmth, compassion, and support and to refrain from making Critical Comments. Finally, for individuals with a chronic illness or those who relapse, intensive individualized interventions and/or family sessions for carers may be needed to specifically mitigate the processes that maintain and perpetuate levels of EE. A stepped-care approach to empirically test a range of carer interventions is highly recommended to identify whether sub-groups of families require more tailored support depending on the stage of the illness.

EE Among Healthcare Providers

EE in paid caregivers of those providing treatment to affected individuals with eating disorders has yet to be investigated, despite the extensive research on unpaid caregivers over the past decade (Treasure & Nazar, 2016). Researchers in psychosis have examined whether the concept of EE is applicable to practitioners working with patients with schizophrenia (Berry, Barrowclough, & Haddock, 2011). According to Berry and colleagues, several salient characteristics (limited experience and knowledge of schizophrenia) in practitioners were associated with negative attributions of affected individuals receiving treatment. Building on this important work, future research is required to understand how practitioner characteristics (age, gender, years of experience, and training) might influence the types of attributions that are assigned to individuals with eating disorders. Future research is further suggested to understand how the emotional climate of an inpatient or day treatment unit may influence patients and patient outcomes.

Exploration of EE in a Range of Dyads

The cognitive interpersonal model of AN (Treasure & Schmidt, 2013) targets problematic patterns of interactions that may lead to treatment resistance in adults with eating disorders. The majority of research has focused on levels of EE in parent and adolescent dyads or the family climate of an adolescent and young adult with an eating disorder (Chapters 2, 3, 4, and 5). As described in Chapter 5, the next generation of research on EE should assess and address levels of EE from those affected with an eating disorder towards their loved ones and other family members, including siblings and partners, who shape the climate of the family.

Treasure and her colleagues (Chapter 7) propose a model that demonstrates how social cognition and interpersonal factors contribute to both risk and maintenance of eating disorders in individuals. Neuroscience shows that people with eating disorders experience impairment in accurately reading facial expressions and/or being overly attuned to threat (Caglar-Nazali et al., 2014). As described in Chapter 7 by Treasure and her colleagues, this body of research further demonstrates that people with eating disorders attend to cues of rejection and avoid socially rewarding ones, with limited opportunities to develop effective communication and problem-solving skills. The majority of research conducted in this area focuses on parents who are carers of individuals with eating disorders. To date, there are no studies describing EE in couples when one person is affected by an eating disorder. Research in depression shows that partners' level of criticism was influenced by the affected individual's depression and readiness for treatment for their illness (Meuwly,

Bodenmann, & Coyne, 2012). Research on couple interventions is highly recommended to target the Critical Comments, accommodations, and warmth in intimate dyads affected by a range of eating disorders.

To date, there is little research examining the influence of EE in parents with eating disorders towards their child's psychosocial development and long-term outcomes. Future research is needed on parental–child dyads when a *parent* has an eating disorder (or other mental health disorder). Research shows that parental depression leads to heightened parental criticism towards children (Rogosch, Cicchetti, & Toth, 2004). Mothers with depression model behavior inhibition to their children and are less likely to demonstrate warmth towards their children (Downey & Coyne, 1990). Research is required to identify how EE in parents with an eating disorder may manifest itself differentially in their interactions with their children based on their children's temperament, gender, and age. This line of research may help shed light on whether mothers with eating disorders respond with varying levels of Criticism and Warmth towards their children of different weight, shape and size, and eating patterns. Do parents with eating disorders exhibit disgust and withdraw from their children when they are eating foods that they typically avoid or binge on? An increased understanding of EE in parents with eating disorders may lead to the development of interventions that could improve outcomes for the affected parent, children, and family as a whole.

The chapter led by Gorrell and Le Grange (Chapter 5) provides a summary of the bidirectional nature of EE between caregivers and affected individuals. Gorrell and Le Grange highlight the need for greater research on patients' experiences of parental EE, patients' own levels of EE, and the interaction between these two processes in predicting treatment outcomes and relapse. Furthermore, this chapter noted the importance of examining levels of EE longitudinally rather than just in the acute phase of the illness. This chapter also called for more research on Warmth and Positive Remarks, which have received minimal attention in the eating disorders research when compared with EOI and criticism (Le Grange, Hoste, Lock, & Bryson, 2011).

Conclusion

For over half a century, EE has remained a relevant and important construct in the field of psychopathology, due to the pioneering work of a number of researchers, including George Brown, Julian Leff, and Christine Vaughn. Although this work was anchored in the study of schizophrenia and depression, over the years EE has been found to be an important and robust prognostic indicator of treatment outcome, treatment dropout, and relapse across a range of medical and psychiatric disorders, including eating disorders. However, much remains unknown about EE in the context of eating disorders. It is our hope that this book will serve to inspire current and future clinicians and researchers to further explore this rich and promising area of study.

References

Altorfer, A., Käsermann, M.-L., & Hirsbrunner, H. (1998). Arousal and communication: 1. The relationship between nonverbal, behavioral, and physiological indices of the stress response. *Journal of Psychophysiology, 12*, 40–59.

Beck, A. T., & Clark, D. A. (1988). Anxiety and depression: An information processing perspective. *Anxiety Research, 1*, 23–36.

Berry, K., Barrowclough, C., & Haddock, G. (2011). The role of expressed emotion in relationships between psychiatric staff and people with a diagnosis of psychosis: A review of the literature. *Schizophrenia Bulletin, 37*, 958–972.

Brown, G. W., Birley, J. L. T., & Wing, J. K. (1972). Influence of family life on the course of schizophrenic disorders: A replication. *British Journal of Psychiatry, 121*, 241–258.

Butzlaff, R. L., & Hooley, J. M. (1998). Expressed emotion and psychiatric relapse: A meta-analysis. *Archives of General Psychiatry, 55*, 547–552.

Caglar-Nazali, H. P., Corfield, F., Cardi, V., Ambwani, S., Leppanen, J., Olabintan, O., . . . Treasure, J. (2014). A systematic review and meta-analysis of "systems for social processes" in eating disorders. *Neuroscience & Biobehavioral Reviews, 42*, 55–92.

Caqueo-Urízar, A., Rus-Calafell, M., Urzúa, A., Escudero, J., & Gutiérrez-Maldonado, J. (2015). The role of family therapy in the management of schizophrenia: Challenges and solutions. *Neuropsychiatric Disease and Treatment, 11*, 145–151.

Christiansen, H., Oades, R. D., Psychogiou, L., Hauffa, B. P., & Sonuga-Barke, E. J. (2010). Does the cortisol response to stress mediate the link between expressed emotion and oppositional defiant disorder in attention deficit hyperactivity disorder. *Behavioral and Brain Functions, 6*, 45.

Davis, K. L., Kahn, R. S., Ko, G., & Davidson, M. (1991). Dopamine in schizophrenia: A review and reconceptualization. *American Journal of Psychiatry, 148*, 1474–1486.

Dimitropoulos, G., Landers, A., Freeman, V., Novick, J., Schmidt, U., & Olmsted, M. (2019). A feasibility study comparing a web-based intervention to a workshop intervention for caregivers of adults with eating disorders. *European Eating Disorders Review*. doi:10.1002/erv.2678

Downey, G., & Coyne, J. C. (1990). Children of depressed parents: An integrative review. *Psychological Bulletin, 108*, 50–76.

Foland-Ross, L. C., & Gotlib, I. H. (2012). Cognitive and neural aspects of information processing in major depressive disorder: An integrative perspective. *Frontiers in Psychology, 3*, 489.

Haigh, R., & Treasure, J. (2003). Investigating the needs of carers in the area of eating disorders: Development of the Carers' Needs Assessment Measure (CaNAM). *European Eating Disorders Review, 11*, 125–141.

Hibbs, E. D., Zahn, T. P., Hamburger, S. D., & Kruesi, M. M. (1992). Parental expressed emotion and psychophysiological reactivity in disturbed and normal children. *British Journal of Psychiatry, 160*, 504–510.
Hibbs, R., Magill, N., Goddard, E., Rhind, C., Raenker, S., Macdonald, P., . . . Treasure, J. (2015). Clinical effectiveness of a skills training intervention for caregivers in improving patient and caregiver health following in-patient treatment for severe anorexia nervosa: Pragmatic randomised controlled trial. *BJPsych Open, 1*, 556–566.
Hooley, J. M., & Gotlib, I. H. (2000). A diathesis-stress conceptualization of expressed emotion and clinical outcome. *Applied & Preventive Psychology, 9*, 135–151.
Hooley, J. M., & Hoffman, P. D. (1999). Expressed emotion and clinical outcome in borderline personality disorder. *American Journal of Psychiatry, 156*, 1557–1562.
Hoste, R. R., Lebow, J., & Le Grange, D. (2015). A bidirectional examination of expressed emotion among families of adolescents with bulimia nervosa. *International Journal of Eating Disorders, 48*, 249–252.
Humphreys, K. L., Watts, E. L., Dennis, E. L., King, L. S., Thompson, P. M., & Gotlib, I. H. (2019). Stressful life events, ADHD symptoms, and brain structure in early adolescence. *Journal of Abnormal Child Psychology, 47*, 421–432.
Jappe, L. M., Frank, G. K. W., Shott, M. E., Rollin, D. H., Pryor, T., Hagman, J. O., . . . Davis, E. (2011). Heightened sensitivity to reward and punishment in anorexia nervosa. *International Journal of Eating Disorders, 44*, 317–324.
Jenkins, J. H., & Karno, M. (1992). The meaning of expressed emotion: Theoretical issues raised by cross-cultural research. *American Journal of Psychiatry, 149*, 9–21.
Le Grange, D., Hoste, R. R., Lock, J., & Bryson, S. W. (2011). Parental expressed emotion of adolescents with anorexia nervosa: Outcome in family-based treatment. *International Journal of Eating Disorders, 44*, 731–734.
Lock, J., & Le Grange, D. (2013). *Treatment manual for anorexia nervosa: A family-based approach* (2nd ed.). New York, NY: Guilford Press.
Meuwly, N., Bodenmann, G., & Coyne, J. C. (2012). The association between partners' expressed emotion and depression: Mediated by patients' dysfunctional attitudes? *Journal of Social and Clinical Psychology, 31*, 690–706.
Millman, Z. B., Weintraub, M. J., & Miklowitz, D. J. (2018). Expressed emotion, emotional distress, and individual and familial history of affective disorder among parents of adolescents with bipolar disorder. *Psychiatry Research, 270*, 656–660.
Morgado, P., Freitas, D., Bessa, J. M., Sousa, N., & Cerqueira, J. J. (2013). Perceived stress in obsessive-compulsive disorder is related with obsessive but not compulsive symptoms. *Frontiers in Psychiatry, 4*, 21.
Pépin, G., & King, R. (2013). Collaborative care skills training workshops: Helping carers cope with eating disorders from the UK to Australia. *Social Psychiatry and Psychiatric Epidemiology, 48*, 805–812.
Peris, T. S., & Miklowitz, D. J. (2015). Parental expressed emotion and youth psychopathology new directions for an old construct. *Child Psychiatry & Human Development, 46*, 863–873.
Rienecke, R. D., Accurso, E. C., Lock, J., & Le Grange, D. (2016). Expressed emotion, family functioning, and treatment outcome for adolescents with anorexia nervosa. *European Eating Disorders Review, 24*, 43–51.
Rienecke, R. D., Lebow, J., Lock, J., & Le Grange, D. (2017). Family profiles of expressed emotion in adolescent patients with anorexia nervosa and their parents. *Journal of Clinical Child & Adolescent Psychology, 46*, 428–436.
Rogosch, F. A., Cicchetti, D., & Toth, S. L. (2004). Expressed emotion in multiple subsystems of the families of toddlers with depressed mothers. *Development and Psychopathology, 16*, 689–709.

Schwarte, R., Timmesfeld, N., Dempfle, A., Krei, M., Egberts, K., Jaite, C., . . . Bühren, K. (2017). Expressed emotions and depressive symptoms in caregivers of adolescents with first-onset anorexia nervosa: A long-term investigation over 2.5 years. *European Eating Disorders Review, 25*, 44–51.
Sturgeon, D., Turpin, G., Kuipers, L., Berkowitz, R., & Leff, J. (1984). Psychophysiological responses of schizophrenic patients to high and low expressed emotion relatives: A follow-up study. *British Journal of Psychiatry, 145*, 62–69.
Tarrier, N., Vaughn, C., Lader, M. H., & Leff, J. P. (1979). Bodily reactions to people and events in schizophrenia. *Archives of General Psychiatry, 36*, 311–315.
Treasure, J., & Nazar, B. P. (2016). Interventions for the carers of patients with eating disorders. *Current Psychiatry Reports, 18*. doi:10.1007/s119250-015-0652-3
Treasure, J., & Schmidt, U. (2013). The cognitive-interpersonal maintenance model of anorexia nervosa revisited: A summary of the evidence for cognitive, socio-emotional and interpersonal predisposing and perpetuating factors. *Journal of Eating Disorders, 1*, 13.
Vaughn, C. E., & Leff, J. P. (1976). The influence of family and social factors on the course of psychiatric illness: A comparison of schizophrenic and depressed neurotic patients. *British Journal of Psychiatry, 129*, 125–137.
Wearden, A. J., Tarrier, N., Barrowclough, C., Zastowny, T. R., & Rahill, A. A. (2000). A review of expressed emotion research in health care. *Clinical Psychology Review, 20*, 633–666.

Index

Note: Page numbers in *italics* indicate a figure and page numbers in **bold** indicate a table on the corresponding page.

ABOS *see* Anorectic Behavior Observation Scale (ABOS)
acceptance-based separated family-based therapy (ASFT) 83
accommodation 118, **124**
ADHD *see* attention deficit/hyperactivity disorder (ADHD)
adolescent-focused therapy (AFT) 81–82
affect regulation processes 45
AFT *see* adolescent-focused therapy (AFT)
alexithymia 47–48, 120
AN *see* anorexia nervosa (AN)
Anorectic Behavior Observation Scale (ABOS) 108
anorexia nervosa (AN) 38–39, 41–42, 62, 67, 69, 76–97, 102–103, 105, 107, 109, 115–119, *117*, 118, 119, 137–138, **142**–**147**, 158–160, 163, 177, 179–181
anxiety 2, 11
appraisals, patient 13
ARFID *see* avoidant/restrictive food intake disorder (ARFID)
ASFT *see* acceptance-based separated family-based therapy (ASFT)
attention bias 120–121
attention deficit/hyperactivity disorder (ADHD) 178
attributional style, caregiver 165–166
avoidance **124**
avoidant/restrictive food intake disorder (ARFID) 177

BDI *see* Beck Depression Inventory (BDI)
BDSEE *see* Brief Dyadic Scale of Expressed Emotion (BDSEE)
Beck Depression Inventory (BDI) 105
BED *see* binge eating disorder (BED)
bias, attention and interpretation 120–121
binge eating disorder (BED) 101, 138, 160–161

BN *see* bulimia nervosa (BN)
borderline personality disorder (BPD) 179
BPD *see* borderline personality disorder (BPD)
Brief Dyadic Scale of Expressed Emotion (BDSEE) 70, 72
Brown, George 1, 33
bulimia nervosa (BN) 39–40, 76, 86, 101–110, 138, **142–147**, 160, 163, 177, 179, 181

Calgary Family Intervention Model (CFIM) 108
Camberwell Family Interview (CFI) 2, 4, 34, 36, 59–65, 67–68, 70–72, 77, 79, 104–105, 149
caregiver(s): attributional style of 165–166; of bulimia nervosa patients, interventions for 108–109; burden and distress among 88–90, 162–163; coping of 164–165; culture and 132; expressed emotion, bidirectional relationship in patient and 90–92; expressed emotions in relationships with, in psychosis 10–12; factors associated with level of expressed emotion 162–167; gender of 166–167; impact on 8–10; psychological distress among 163; reactions to expressed emotion reactions of 119; sleep quality in 10; warmth of 13–14
CC *see* Critical Comments (CC)
CFI *see* Camberwell Family Interview (CFI)
CFIM *see* Calgary Family Intervention Model (CFIM)
CFT *see* conjoint family therapy (CFT)
cognition, social 119–121
cognitive interpersonal model 116–122, *117*
cognitive reappraisal 15, 17, 19, 21–22, 24
cognitive reframing 15, 17, 19, 22, 24
communication support 122–125
compliance, treatment 39–40
conjoint family therapy (CFT) 80–81, 92
coping 12–13; caregiver 164–165
Critical Comments (CC) 34–35, 60–62, 67, 77–80, 83, 87, 89, 94, 105, 108, 118, 130–131, 156–157, 161, 166, 168, 176, 178–179, 183
culture: caregivers and 132; critical comments and 130–131; defined 129; eating disorders and 136–140; emotional overinvolvement and 131–132; familial criticism and 130–131

depression 2, 9, 12, 60–61, 104–106
diabetes 2, 10
dolphin metaphor **123**
duration of illness 159–160

Eating Disorder Inventory (EDI) 105, 138–139
eating disorders (EDs): culture and 136–140; expressed emotion and 38–43; severity of 39
ECHO *see* Experienced Carers Helping Others (ECHO)
EDI *see* Eating Disorder Inventory (EDI)
EDs *see* eating disorders (EDs)
Emotional Overinvolvement (EOI) 10, 12–14, 34–35, 42, 60, 64, 68–69, 83–84, 86–88, 91, 119, 131–132, 156–157, 166, 168, 178
emotion regulation *44*
enabling **124**
engagement, treatment 39–40
EOI *see* Emotional Overinvolvement (EOI)
epilepsy 2
ethnic differences, in expressed emotion 109
Experienced Carers Helping Others (ECHO) 94, 125
expressed emotion (EE): across stages of illness 180–181; among healthcare providers 181–182; assessment of 58–73; bidirectional relationship

in patient and caregiver 90–92; as "black box" 177; bulimia nervosa and 104–107; in caregiving relationships in psychosis 10–12; changes in parental 92–94; cultural differences in 129–150, **142–147**; defined 58; and duration of illness 159–160; eating disorders and 38–43; ethnic differences in 109; factors associated with high *vs.* low 156–169; future directions in 176–184; in historical perspective 33–34; history of concept 1–2; integrated theoretical framework for 180; interactional nature of 36–38; low, in families 47–48; measurement of 34–36, 58; mechanisms of action in 177–180; parent and patient characteristics associated with 85–90; patient 161–162; patient factors in 157–162; in range of dyads 182–184; symptom severity and 158–159; as toxic family stress 178–179; treatment outcome and 40–41, 76–85; treatment response and 40; as treatment target 41–43
Expressed Emotion Index 129

families: bulimia nervosa and 107–108; low expressed emotion in 47–48; stress in 37; working with 14–16
Family Attitude Scale (FAS) 70–71
family-based treatment (FBT) 41, 81, 83–85, 115–116
Family Emotional Involvement and Criticism Scale (FEICS) 70, 72
Family Environment Scale (FES) 105
family factors, in level of expressed emotion 167–168
family interventions in psychosis (FIp) 14–15, 25
Family Problems Questionnaire 104
Family Questionnaire (FQ) 68–69, 83, 92, 94–95, 106, 108
family relationships, positive 13–14
family support, psychosis and 8
FAS *see* Family Attitude Scale (FAS)
FBT *see* family-based treatment (FBT)
FEICS *see* Family Emotional Involvement and Criticism Scale (FEICS)
FES *see* Family Environment Scale (FES)
FIp *see* family interventions in psychosis (FIp)
Five-Minute Speech Sample (FMSS) 34–35, 42, 63–65, 67
FMSS *see* Five-Minute Speech Sample (FMSS)
FQ *see* Family Questionnaire (FQ)
fragmentation **124**
Frankl, Viktor 121

gender: caregiver, and level of expressed emotion 166–167; parent, treatment outcome and 84–85
genetics 43, *44*, 122

healthcare providers, expressed emotion among 181–182
herd of elephants metaphor **123**
Hostility (H) 34, 77–78, 118, 122, 156, 166, 178

illness beliefs 12–13
interactional, expressed emotion as 36–38, 43
interpretation bias 120–121
interviews, semi-structured 59–65
isolation 115

journal, positive qualities 20, 22, 24

kangaroo metaphor **123**

LEE *see* Level of Expressed Emotion (LEE) Scale
Leff, Julian 1–2, 33
Level of Expressed Emotion (LEE) Scale 66–68, 71–72, 106, 108, 148–149

life expectancy 8
loneliness 115

major depressive disorder (MDD) 104–105; *see also* depression
maladaptive interpersonal reactions 122–125, **123–124**
MDD *see* major depressive disorder (MDD)
mentalization 37, 45
mother, schizophrenogenic 2

NATs *see* negative automatic thoughts (NATs)
negative automatic thoughts (NATs) 18–19, 21, 23
neurobiology 43–48

ostrich metaphor **124**
outcome, treatment 40–41, 58, 76–85
overprotection 119, 122, **123**

parent-focused therapy (PFT) 41, 81–82, 84
patient appraisals 13
PFT *see* parent-focused therapy (PFT)
positive family relationships 13–14
Positive Remarks (PR) 34, 60, 95, 141, 156, 161, 167
PR *see* Positive Remarks (PR)
psychological distress, caregiver 163
psychosis: expressed emotions in caregiving relationships in 10–12; family support and 8; negative emotional sequelae of perceived expressed emotion in 16–24; working with families in 14–16

questionnaires 65–72

regulation, emotion *44*
rehearsal 16
rejection sensitivity 43–44
response, treatment 40
rhinoceros metaphor **124**
role-play 16–17, 19–20, 22, 24
Rutter, Michael 33

SCFI *see* Standardized Clinical Family Interview (SCFI)
schizoaffective disorder 18–23
schizophrenia 1, 10, 23–24, 33–34, 103, 132, 178–180
schizophrenia spectrum disorders 7
schizophrenogenic mother 2
self-esteem 11, 15–16
self-report scales 65–72
semi-structured interviews 59–65
separated family therapy (SFT) 80–81, 92
SFT *see* separated family therapy (SFT)
SIAB *see* Structured Interview for Anorexia and Bulimia Nervosa (SIAB)
"sick role" 119
skill-sharing interventions 125
sleep, in caregivers 10
social cognition 119–121
Standardized Clinical Family Interview (SCFI) 61–63, 65, 72, 78, 82, 85, 105, 107, 109, 149
St Bernard metaphor **123**
stress 37
Structured Interview for Anorexia and Bulimia Nervosa (SIAB) 105

terrier metaphor **124**
therapeutic alliance 46
threat sensitivity 43, *44*, 120–121
toxic family stress 178–179
treatment compliance 39–40
treatment engagement 39–40
treatment outcome 40–41, 58, 76–85
treatment response 40

Vaughn, Christine 1–2, 33

Warmth (W) 34, 60, 87, 95, 118, 141, 156, 161

Made in the USA
Monee, IL
12 November 2026

d45af355-c022-4ae7-a950-d67b2ecef33aR01